MCQs for MRCP Part 1
General Medicine

Michael J Ford MBChB (Hons) MD FRCP (Edin)

Consultant Physician and Honorary Senior Lecturer
Western General Hospital, Edinburgh, UK

Ian B Wilkinson MA BM MRCP(UK)

Senior Lecturer and Honorary Consultant Physician
Clinical Pharmacology Unit
Addenbrooke's Hospital, Cambridge UK

THIRD EDITION

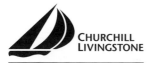

CHURCHILL
LIVINGSTONE

EDINBURGH LONDON NEW YORK OXFORD PHILADELPHIA
ST LOUIS SYDNEY TORONTO 2004

CHURCHILL LIVINGSTONE   at Derby Library
An imprint of Elsevier Limited

© Longman Group Limited 1986
© Longman Group Limited 1995
© Harcourt Publishers Limited 1999

© 2004, Elsevier Limited. All rights reserved.

First published 1986
Second edition 1995
Third edition 2004

ISBN 0-443-07361-9

British Library Cataloguing in Publication Data
A catalogue record for this book is available from the British Library

Library of Congress Cataloging in Publication Data
A catalog record for this book is available from the Library of Congress

Notice
Medical knowledge is constantly changing. Standard safety precautions must be followed, but as new research and clinical experience broaden our knowledge, changes in treatment and drug therapy may become necessary or appropriate. Readers are advised to check the most current product information provided by the manufacturer of each drug to be administered to verify the recommended dose, the method and duration of administration, and contraindications. It is the responsibility of the practitioner, relying on experience and knowledge of the patient, to determine dosages and the best treatment for each individual patient. Neither the Publisher nor the authors assumes any liability for any injury and/or damage to persons or property arising from this publication.
The Publisher

ELSEVIER SCIENCE

your source for books,
journals and multimedia
in the health sciences

www.elsevierhealth.com

The publisher's policy is to use paper manufactured from sustainable forests

Printed in China

MCQs for
MRCP Part 1
General Medicine

Commissioning Editors: Laurence Hunter and Ellen Green
Project Development Manager: Siân Jarman
Project Manager: Frances Affleck
Designer: Erik Bigland

Preface

The MRCP(UK) Part 1 examination is the first substantial hurdle for aspiring physicians and many young doctors approach this with considerable apprehension. We have addressed this problem in the contents of this book which aims to help candidates prepare themselves appropriately for this examination.

The book is organized in chapters with appropriate numbers of 'best of five' multiple choice questions similar to those in the MRCP(UK) Part 1 examination (General Medicine). Only paediatric questions relevant to adolescent medicine have been included. Many new questions in clinical science and practice have been introduced and the format of the questions aligned with the new format of the revised MRCP(UK) Part 1 examination.

We are particularly grateful to Dr David Matthews, author of the 1995 edition, for all of his hard work, enthusiasm and commitment.

Edinburgh and Cambridge   M.J.F.
                                                               I.B.W.

v

Contents

Preparation for the MRCP(UK) Part 1 examination

In preparing for the examination, there is no substitute for a detailed study of all areas of clinical medicine. For many, this cannot be achieved without at least 3 months of regular reading prior to the MRCP(UK) Part 1 examination. Some find it useful to meet in groups and prepare topics for discussion, including MCQs, beforehand. In this way, areas of difficulty in understanding can often be resolved. In addition, prospective candidates will feel more confident that they are ready to take the examination. If, however, after enrolling for the examination, a candidate does not feel adequately prepared, he/she would be better advised to withdraw from the examination, saving time and money, rather than proceeding in a speculative way on the off chance of passing the examination.

Reading a standard textbook of medicine is important in preparation for the examination, and in this regard, the textbooks of medicine by Souhami and Moxham, Kumar and Clark and Davidson's *Principles in Practice* are each as appropriate. Larger textbooks, such as Harrison's *Principles of Internal Medicine* or *The Oxford Textbook of Medicine* are useful to clarify reference items, but too large and comprehensive to be appropriate day-to-day manuals. *The British National Formulary*, published twice yearly, is an excellent educational resource in revising clinical pharmacology and therapeutics. It is well worth reading, particularly the text at the beginning of each section.

MRCP(UK) PART 1 SYLLABUS (GENERAL MEDICINE)

The syllabus for the MRCP(UK) Part 1 examination is available from the MRCP(UK) Central Office and provides details of the methods used to set and assess the examination. It gives information to candidates wishing to know about the subjects covered in the examination. An interactive CD is available containing six past MRCP(UK) Part 1 examination papers from 1997 and 1998. The interactive CD allows candidates to sit the papers set for each diet, produce their own test papers covering one or more topics or have an examination set by the computer program. Candidates can also indicate their degree of confidence in their answers ('Educated guess' or 'Complete guess').

MRCP(UK) PART 1 EXAMINATION

The MRCP(UK) Part 1 examination consists of two papers. Both papers comprise 100 multiple choice questions in the *'best of five'* format, where a candidate must choose the single best answer from five possible answers. The questions have been devised to test candidates' knowledge of a wide range of common and important disorders in general medicine in typical encounters including outpatient and inpatient settings as outlined in MRCP (UK) published syllabus.

Overall composition of the MRCP(UK) Part 1 by specialty:

Cardiology	15
Clinical sciences* (see below)	25
Clinical pharmacology, therapeutics and toxicology	20
Gastroenterology and hepatology	15
Clinical haematology and oncology	15
Infectious and sexually-transmitted diseases	15
Endocrinology	15
Nephrology	8
Neurology	15
Respiratory medicine	15
Rheumatology	15
Psychiatry	15
Dermatology	8
Ophthalmology	4

*

Cell/membrane biology	2
Clinical anatomy	3
Clinical biochemistry	4
Clinical physiology	4
Genetics	3
Immunology	4
Epidemiology and statistics	5

MRCP(UK) PART 1 EXAMINATION

Purpose

The purpose of the MRCP(UK) Part 1 examination is to identify those physicians in training who, having satisfied the entry criteria, possess a broad knowledge and understanding of basic clinical science as well as common and important disorders.

Aims

The aims of the MRCP(UK) Part 1 examination are to test the acquisition of medical knowledge as outlined in the MRCP(UK) Part 1 syllabus, to measure candidates' abilities to apply medical knowledge of the common and important topics and to make appropriate clinical judgements.

EXAMPLES OF THE STYLE AND FORMAT OF MRCP(UK) PART 1 MCQs

1   **A 55-year-old man with hypertension presents with exertional chest pain which occurs after walking uphill and which has persisted unchanged over the previous 3 months. Which ONE of the following statements is TRUE?**
   A   nitrates should improve exercise tolerance by reducing the venous return
   B   cardioselective beta-blockers are likely to be more effective than non-cardioselective beta-blockers in preventing the progression of angina
   C   digoxin therapy should be introduced to improve exercise tolerance
   D   calcium-channel blockers will reduce the risk of sudden death
   E   beta-blockade does not prevent the tachycardia induced by nitrate therapy

Answer key: A

2   **An elderly diabetic patient is admitted unconscious, having been seen in excellent health 4 hours previously. Which ONE of the following clinical features suggests that the impairment of consciousness is more likely to be attributable to hypoglycaemia than diabetic ketoacidosis?**
   A   systemic hypotension
   B   extensor plantar responses
   C   deep sighing respirations
   D   dry skin
   E   abdominal pain

Answer key: B

APPROACH TO MCQ EXAMINATIONS

In tackling multiple-choice questions, there are certain helpful ground rules, and these include:

Read the question very carefully

We all misread words occasionally, particularly when under stress. It is easy to see how chlorpropamide and chlorpromazine can be confused in the context of an examination.

Ask yourself why the question is being posed in this way

This can be a useful way of approaching questions, because what appears to be an obvious question with an obvious answer may be less obvious on careful re-reading. The wording of the question has been designed to help you avoid an erroneous interpretation of the question, not to trick you. For instance, the answer to the question 'Which of the

3

following features favour a diagnosis of myocardial infarction rather than acute pulmonary embolism?' is very different from the answer to the question 'Which of the following features favour a diagnosis of acute pulmonary embolism rather than myocardial infarction?'

Logical reasoning is better than blind guesswork

Even the best informed do not know all the answers. It is important that candidates remember that there is no negative marking and any errors you make will not be penalized. It is often possible to deduce an answer by reasoned and careful logic, even when one cannot recall reading the answer to such a question in any text. The wording in some multiple-choice questions may appear difficult to those who are inexperienced at MCQs. The words 'always', 'never', or 'invariably' are rarely seen in an MCQ examination, as they beg the answer 'false'; the practice of medicine does not often deal with such degrees of certainty. Similarly, the words 'can' or 'may' are unusual in MCQs given that most things are possible in medicine. When such words are seen, therefore, the correct answer to the question is more often false than true. The word 'pathognomonic' means that the occurrence of a sign or symptom is 100% specific to the disease stated and never occurs in the absence of the disease. If the words 'frequently', 'commonly' or 'usually' are used, this means that the symptoms or signs stated are a feature in at least 50% of instances. When the words 'characteristically' or 'typically' are used, this means that such symptoms or signs may not occur in the majority of instances, but when they do occur, they are of considerable diagnostic or therapeutic significance. Finally, the word 'recognized' means that the occurrence of a sign or symptom has been reported in the medical literature, though it may be a rare event.

HOW TO COMPLETE THE ANSWER SHEETS

Candidates indicate their answers to the questions by completing answer sheets, which are machine-read by an optical mark reader (OMR). The output from the OMR is processed by computer and marks are allocated according to the candidate's responses, scores are calculated and statistical data derived relating to individual questions: this information is produced in printed form for the MRCP(UK) Part 1 Examining Board. As the completed answer sheets are computer marked, you must comply fully with the instructions given on each answer sheet, otherwise answer sheets may be rejected by the machine or your intention misinterpreted. Use only the pencil (Grade 2B) supplied in the examination. Answers in ink or in a different grade of pencil cannot be read by the optical mark reader. First, identify yourself; write your surname and initials in the boxes provided. Next, complete your examination number using the appropriate rectangles.

The answer sheets for the Part 1 MRCP(UK) contain rows of rectangles for each question. Indicate the single correct answer, in accordance with the instructions given on the examination paper. Indicate the best answer from the five possible answers given, by pencilling in the

4

appropriate rectangle. If you do not know the answer, either make a reasoned guess or leave it blank as there is no negative marking. Erase an answer by using the rubber eraser provided. Avoid making too many erasures on the answer sheet by recording your choices in the question book in the first instance, before transferring them to the answer sheet. Remember to allow sufficient time to do so, as extra time will not be allowed. Do not fold or crease your answer sheet as this may alter the accuracy of the optical scanning of your answers.

MRCP(UK) PART 1 SCORING AND ASSESSMENT

Each question in the entire MRCP(UK) Part 1 examination is criterion referenced and assesses a candidate's performance in relation to an external standard of performance (pass mark) set by the examiners. A single pass mark is applied in relation to candidates' overall performance from both papers. No mark is deducted for any wrong answer and one mark (+1) is awarded for each correct answer. No marks are awarded or deducted if the question is either left unanswered or more than one answer per question is recorded. There is a charge of £100 if a candidate requests that their examination is re-marked, which is refundable if an error is identified. Examination scripts are held for 1 year only. Any allegation of academic or professional misconduct that is sustained against a candidate is likely to be reported to employers and the relevant professional bodies such as the UK General Medical Council. Candidates who fail badly may be recommended to defer re-entry for one examination.

MRCP(UK) EXAMINATION: FURTHER INFORMATION

The MRCP(UK) Central Office provide candidates with relevant information about the MRCP(UK) examination and produces useful publications including the syllabus and a selection of questions previously used in the MRCP(UK) examination. The MRCP(UK) Central Office web site is at http://www.mrcpuk.org.

MRCP(UK) PART 1 EXAMINATION SCHEDULE

The MRCP(UK) Part 1 examination consists of two papers each comprising 100 MCQs and lasting 3 hours.

09.30	Report to the examination hall		
10.00	**Paper 1**	**100 'Best of Five' MCQs**	**3 hours**
13.00–14.15	Lunch break		
14.15	Report to the examination hall		
14.30	**Paper 2**	**100 'Best of Five' MCQs**	**3 hours**
17.30	Examination ends		

5

1

Cardiology

QUESTIONS

1.1 Which ONE of the following is MOST likely to be found in a patient with longstanding constrictive pericarditis?
A A wide pulse pressure
B A rise in systolic pressure on inspiration
C Pulsus alternans
D A fall in venous pressure on inspiration
E Ascites

1.2 A 54-year-old male, non-smoker, presents with chest pain. Which ONE of the following features MOST suggests a non-cardiac aetiology?
A A fall in the ejection fraction on exercise echocardiography
B Pain occurring at the start of exercise which then improves during exercise
C Pain relieved by glyceryl trinitrate within 5 minutes
D A normal resting ECG
E Up-sloping ST segment depression occurring during exercise testing

1.3 A 46-year-old woman presents with hypertension. The blood pressure (BP) is 170/108 mmHg, plasma creatinine 190 μmol/L and there is marked left ventricular hypertrophy on the resting ECG. The plasma renin activity is <10 mU/L. She is on no medication other than the combined contraceptive pill. Which ONE of the following statements is TRUE?
A Blood pressure control should lead to regression of left ventricular hypertrophy
B Angiotensin converting enzyme (ACE) inhibitor therapy is contraindicated
C Bendroflumethiazide (bendrofluazide) would be an appropriate choice of antihypertensive agent
D 'White coat' hypertension is a likely possibility
E Oestrogen-containing contraceptive therapy is not contraindicated

1.4 Which ONE of the following abnormalities is MOST likely to be found in a patient diagnosed with syndrome X (metabolic syndrome)?
A hypouricaemia
B hypercholesterolaemia
C haematuria
D hypoinsulinaemia
E hypertriglyceridaemia

1.5 A 58-year-old man who suffered a myocardial infarction 5 years ago presents to the outpatient clinic with tiredness, worsening shortness of breath on exercise, and swollen ankles. Anterior wall hypokinesia is present on echocardiography and the ejection fraction is 40%. Which ONE of the following drug therapies is MOST likely to improve survival?
A Furosemide (frusemide)
B Digoxin
C Isosorbide mononitrate
D Spironolactone
E Verapamil

1.6 Which ONE of the following statements about disorders associated with a bicuspid aortic valve is TRUE?
A The finding occurs more often in females than males
B No association with an abnormal origin to the coronary arteries
C No association with coarctation of the aorta
D A decreased risk of aortic dissection
E An increased risk of endocarditis

1.7 Which ONE of the following statements concerning atrial myxomas is TRUE?
A They are usually found to be malignant on histopathology
B They are the commonest benign tumour in adolescents
C They are most often located in the right atrium
D Often produce thromboembolic events
E Typically associated with a soft first heart sound

1.8 A 67-year-old Caucasian man presents within 4 hours of the onset of crushing, central chest pain. The ECG findings indicate 3 mm ST elevation in the anterior chest leads. Which ONE of the following plasma concentrations is MOST likely to be elevated at presentation?
A Creatinine kinase–MB fraction
B Lactate dehydrogenase
C Troponin I
D Aspartate transaminase
E Troponin T

1.9 **A 76-year-old woman with no significant past medical history is found to be asymptomatically hypertensive. Which ONE of the following statements is TRUE?**
A   Both systolic and diastolic pressures are likely to be elevated
B   Plasma renin is likely to be elevated
C   Secondary hypertension is more likely than in younger patients
D   Treatment of the high BP should reduce the risk of heart failure
E   Treatment of the high BP is unlikely to reduce the risk of stroke significantly

1.10 **Which ONE of the following cardiac findings in an asymptomatic subject requires permanent endocardial pacing?**
A   Intermittent second degree AV block
B   Previous history of recurrent vasovagal syncope
C   Left bundle branch block occurring after myocardial infarction
D   Sick sinus syndrome
E   Third degree AV block following coronary artery bypass surgery

1.11 **A 76-year-old woman presents with a history of syncopal episodes and on echocardiography, she is found to have severe aortic stenosis. Which ONE of the following features is MOST likely to be found on examination?**
A   Pulsus bisferiens
B   A widely split second heart sound
C   A thrill over the right anterior second intercostal space
D   A wide pulse pressure
E   A pan-systolic murmur

1.12 **In a patient presenting with a supraventricular tachycardia, which ONE of the following is LEAST likely to be responsible?**
A   Mitral valve prolapse
B   Lown–Ganong–Levine syndrome
C   Flecainide therapy
D   Lange–Nielsen syndrome
E   Digoxin toxicity

1.13 **A 24-year-old man is admitted to hospital having collapsed. He has a previous history of blackouts which had been attributed to vasovagal syncope. Clinical examination was unremarkable and the resting ECG was normal except for a prolonged QT interval. Which ONE of the following suggests the MOST likely cause of the syncopal episodes?**
A   Use of beta blocker therapy
B   Serum potassium 5.6 mmol/L
C   Family history of premature sudden death
D   Congenital lymphoedema of the lower limbs
E   Resting tachycardia

1.14 Which ONE of the following features suggests an alternative or additional diagnosis to that of severe mitral stenosis?
A Right ventricular hypertrophy
B Left ventricular dilatation
C Dilated left atrium
D Tricuspid regurgitation
E Absence of a diastolic murmur at rest

1.15 At an insurance medical examination, a 50-year-old male is found to be a heavy smoker with a blood pressure of 170/108 mmHg, body mass index 37, serum cholesterol 7.5 mmol/L and HDL-cholesterol 1.3 mmol/L. Which ONE of the following measures is likely to have the greatest impact on reducing his cardiovascular risk?
A Reducing his blood pressure to 140/85 mmHg
B Reducing his total cholesterol by 1.5 mmol/L
C Stopping smoking
D Taking aspirin 75 mg daily
E Losing 8 kg in weight

1.16 In a patient with a wide-complex tachycardia, which ONE of the following ECG findings MOST suggests a supraventricular tachycardia?
A AV dissociation
B Negative chest lead QRS concordance
C QRS axis −60° to −180°
D Fusion beats
E QRS duration 140 milliseconds

1.17 Which ONE of the following is the LEAST LIKELY to be responsible for the finding of impaired left ventricular filling observed on echocardiography?
A Hypertension
B Hypertrophic cardiomyopathy
C Constrictive pericarditis
D Chronic alcohol intake
E Amyloidosis

1.18 A-20-year old is found to have hypertrophic cardiomyopathy on echocardiography. Which ONE of the following disorders suggests that the echocardiographic changes are likely to be due to an additional and unrelated diagnosis?
A Friedreich's ataxia
B Fabry's disease
C Noonan's syndrome
D Pompe's disease
E Devic's syndrome

1.19 **Which ONE of the following findings is most likely to be found in a 30-year-old woman presenting with an acute myocarditis?**
A   Shortness of breath at rest
B   Sinus bradycardia
C   ST segment depression
D   A pericardial effusion on echocardiography
E   A raised serum lactate dehydrogenase level

1.20 **Which ONE of the following features suggests an alternative diagnosis to that of patent ductus arteriosus?**
A   Prominent vascular markings on a chest radiograph
B   Disappearance of the continuous supraclavicular murmur in the supine position
C   A collapsing pulse
D   Right bundle branch block
E   A mid-diastolic murmur in the mitral area

1.21 **On auscultation, a patient is found to have splitting of the second heart sound which increases during expiration. Which ONE of the following disorders suggests that an alternative diagnosis is likely to be present to explain the finding?**
A   Severe hypertension
B   Right bundle branch block
C   Acute unstable angina
D   Aortic stenosis
E   Hypertrophic obstructive cardiomyopathy

1.22 **Which ONE of the following statements about Kawasaki disease is TRUE?**
A   It is more common in girls
B   The incidence in Japan is decreasing
C   Cervical lymphadenopathy is rare
D   Aneurysms are restricted to the coronary arteries
E   Polymorphous exanthema is typical

1.23 **Which ONE of the following statements about hyperlipoproteinaemia is TRUE?**
A   The children of patients with familial type IIa hyperlipoproteinaemia have a 25% chance of inheriting the trait
B   Chylomicrons consist primarily of cholesterol
C   Plasma cholesterol is reduced in the nephrotic syndrome
D   Long-term gemfibrozil therapy decreases the incidence of cardiac events
E   Plasma cholesterol decreases with age

1.24 **A 28-year-old man presents with a fever and breathlessness and is found to have a diastolic murmur along the left sternal edge. The echocardiogram reveals evidence of significant left ventricular dysfunction and aortic regurgitation with vegetations on the aortic valve. Which ONE of the following statements concerning the investigation and management is TRUE?**

A Alpha-haemolytic *streptococci* are likely to be present on blood cultures

B Tetracycline therapy is indicated prior to the results of blood cultures

C Diffuse glomerulonephritis usually leads to irreversible renal failure

D Valve replacement should be deferred until 4 weeks of antibiotic therapy is given

E Blood cultures are unlikely to be positive except during peaks of pyrexia

1.25 **In a patient with tricuspid incompetence, which ONE of the following findings is the MOST likely to be present?**

A Giant 'a' waves in the neck veins

B A soft pulmonary component to the second heart sound

C Evidence of a right ventricular heave

D An increased risk of pulmonary embolism

E A murmur which decreases with inspiration

1.26 **Which ONE of the following statements about a 40-year-old man presenting with upper limb hypertension and rib notching is TRUE?**

A Constriction of the aorta is most likely to be proximal to the left subclavian artery

B An association with pulmonary stenosis would be an expected finding

C Marfan's syndrome is a recognized association

D A to-and-fro continuous murmur is characteristic of the anomaly

E There is likely to be an increased risk of cerebrovascular accidents

1.27 **Which ONE of the following statements about the electrocardiogram is TRUE?**

A Hypokalaemia produces flattened T waves

B Right ventricular hypertrophy causes an anticlockwise rotation

C Pathological Q waves are usually an early feature of acute infarction

D A QT interval of 500 milliseconds is normal, given a heart rate 80 beats/min

E Mobitz type II AV block shows progressive lengthening of the PR interval

1.28 **In a man presenting with acute chest pain and ECG evidence of acute myocardial infarction, which ONE of the following features indicates a poorer prognosis?**
A Atrial fibrillation at onset
B Ventricular fibrillation occurring on day 5 post-infarction
C Left ventricular ejection fraction in range 40–50
D Patient aged 75 or over
E Inferior rather than an anterior infarction

1.29 **Which ONE of the following statements about the cardiac silhouette on a routine chest X-ray is TRUE?**
A Left atrial size can be accurately assessed
B The cardio-thoracic ratio is usually abnormal in right ventricular hypertrophy
C The cardio-thoracic ratio is typically increased in chronic hypoadrenalism
D Estimated LV size correlates poorly with the severity of hypertensive heart disease
E The pulmonary arteries are often prominent in normal adolescents

1.30 **In the assessment of a cardiac catheterization study, which ONE of the following statements is TRUE?**
A A gradient of 20 mmHg across the aortic valve usually indicates severe stenosis
B Pulmonary artery oxygen saturation is independent of the cardiac output
C The mortality from coronary angiography is approximately 5%
D In constrictive pericarditis, end-diastolic pressures are not equal in both ventricles
E A left ventricular end-diastolic pressure of 25 mmHg indicates a myocardial abnormality in the absence of valve disease

1.31 **In atrial tachyarrhythmias, which ONE of the following statements is TRUE?**
A The delta wave in Wolff–Parkinson–White syndrome is due to myocardial activation via an additional conduction pathway
B Ventricular pacing is the best way to control atrial tachycardias
C Atrial fibrillation excludes the diagnosis of Wolff–Parkinson–White syndrome
D Polyuria suggests a ventricular rather than a supraventricular focus
E Atrial tachycardias are rarely as distressing to the patient as ventricular tachycardias

1.32 Routine auscultation of a young, asymptomatic marathon runner at an insurance medical examination reveals a systolic murmur. The murmur is best heard between the left sternal edge and the apex without obvious radiation to the neck or axilla. Which ONE of the following statements about the murmur is TRUE?

A The murmur is likely to be due to a bicuspid aortic valve

B If the murmur radiates to the third left interspace, tricuspid incompetence is likely

C The severity of mitral incompetence is best assessed by pulmonary wedge pressures

D A loud fourth heart sound suggests severe mitral incompetence

E Mitral valve prolapse is the likeliest explanation

1.33 Which ONE of the following statements about congenital ventricular septal defects (VSD), is TRUE?

A In Eisenmenger syndrome, there is a left- to-right shunt

B A large VSD usually closes spontaneously

C If endocarditis develops, the left ventricular cavity is usually involved

D The murmur typically radiates to the carotids

E The defect typically involves the membranous part of the septum

1.34 An elderly hypertensive man presents with a 2-hour history of tearing, central chest pain radiating to his back. The ECG and plasma troponin are both normal. Which ONE of the following is MOST consistent with a diagnosis of aortic dissection?

A The presence of a purely systolic murmur suggesting aortic stenosis

B Pain which increases gradually over several hours after onset

C Persistent bradycardia

D Absence of any past history of hypertension

E Pleural effusion on chest X-ray

1.35 A 22-year-old is admitted with a fever and arthropathy. Which ONE of the following features suggests an alternative diagnosis to that of rheumatic fever?

A Recent group A beta-haemolytic streptococcal infection

B A short rumbling diastolic murmur

C Erythema marginatum sparing the face

D An elevated ESR

E Symmetrical, small joint polyarthropathy

1.36 In which ONE of the following disorders would the development of a congestive cardiomyopathy suggest the presence of an alternative, unrelated diagnosis?

A Thyrotoxicosis

B Chronic alcohol abuse

C Viral myocarditis

D Advanced HIV disease

E X-linked muscular dystrophy

   E X-linked muscular dystrophy

1.37 **In which ONE of the following disorders is the development of pulmonary hypertension primarily due to an increase in pulmonary blood flow?**
   A Chronic bronchitis and emphysema
   B Mitral stenosis
   C Multiple pulmonary emboli
   D Fibrosing alveolitis
   E Ostium primum atrial septal defect

1.38 **A 45-year-old man is being considered for coronary artery bypass surgery. Which ONE of the following criteria is the MOST appropriate indication for surgery rather than percutaneous coronary intervention?**
   A Asymptomatic airline pilot with an abnormal exercise ECG
   B Symptomatic patient with left main coronary artery stenosis
   C Symptomatic but untreated angina
   D Triple vessel disease with severe left ventricular failure
   E Symptoms of angina with normal coronary angiography

1.39 **A 24-year-old woman presents with a history of episodic breathlessness and palpitation associated with weight gain, mild hypertension and painless diarrhoea. On clinical examination, she appears Cushingoid and tremulous. The electrocardiogram is normal. Which ONE of the following is the MOST likely cause?**
   A Excessive consumption of coffee
   B Phaeochromocytoma
   C Alcohol abuse
   D Carcinoid syndrome
   E Wolff–Parkinson–White syndrome

1.40 **A patient is seen in the review clinic after having had a mitral valve replacement with a Starr–Edwards ball valve prosthetic valve. Which ONE of the following statements is TRUE?**
   A The patient is no longer at risk from endocarditis
   B The left atrial size returns to normal
   C X-ray screening is useful in assessing postoperative valve function
   D A reduction in the intensity of the valve click is unlikely to be of any significance
   E Concomitant omeprazole therapy will reduce the efficacy of warfarin therapy

ANSWERS

1.1   A ✗ Pulse pressure narrows
      B ✗ Systolic pressure falls
      C ✗
      D ✗ Venous pressure rises
      E ✔

1.2   A ✗
      B ✗ Typical of 'first effort angina'
      C ✗
      D ✗
      E ✔ Ischaemia is indicated by down sloping or horizontal ST segment depression

1.3   A ✔
      B ✗ Treatment with an ACE inhibitor helps preserve renal function. Renal artery stenosis should be excluded but is unlikely with the low plasma renin activity
      C ✗ Thiazide diuretics are ineffective in subjects with renal impairment
      D ✗ End-organ damage due to hypertension is present
      E ✗ Most women experience a small rise in BP on starting the pill. However, this rise is exaggerated in some individuals

1.4   A ✗
      B ✗ Total cholesterol may be normal but HDL is usually reduced
      C ✗ Proteinuria may occur and is associated with an increased mortality
      D ✗ 'Insulin resistance syndrome'
      E ✔

1.5   A ✗ May reduce symptoms
      B ✗ Improves symptoms even if not in AF, but no change in survival
      C ✗ No evidence that nitrates alone increase survival
      D ✔ The RALES study
      E ✗ Relatively contraindicated in CCF

1.6   A ✗ Male:female ratio is 4:1
      B ✗
      C ✗ 50% of coarctations are found in association with a BAV
      D ✗ Increased risk of dissection
      E ✔ A bicuspid valve can be found in 20–25% of cases of aortic valve endocarditis

1.7 A ✘ Usually benign tumours
B ✘ Rhabdomyoma accounts for ~50% of benign tumours at this age
C ✘ Over 80% are in the left atrium
D ✔ Up to 60% of cases
E ✘ Usually a loud first or second heart sound, and holosystolic and diastolic murmurs

1.8 A ✔ Elevated after 4–6 hours and peaks at 12 hours
B ✘ Elevated after 12 hours
C ✘ Elevated after 6–12 hours and remains elevated for 7–10 days
D ✘ Elevated after 12 hours
E ✘ Elevated after 6–12 hours and remains elevated for 7–10 days

1.9 A ✘ Isolated systolic hypertension accounts for ~70% of all cases
B ✘ Renin falls with age, and unless there is renal artery stenosis or concomitant drug therapy (e.g. thiazide diuretics), is usually low in the elderly
C ✘ Secondary hypertension is most commonly detected in young subjects with resistant hypertension
D ✔ The risk of heart failure can be reduced by 30–40%
E ✘ The risk of stroke is reduced by ~33% and MI by 25%

1.10 A ✘ Persistent, symptomatic second or third degree AV block
B ✘
C ✘
D ✘ May improve survival if bradycardia limits exercise tolerance
E ✔

1.11 A ✘ Indicates mixed aortic valve disease without severe stenosis
B ✘ Usually single second sound, or reverse splitting
C ✔
D ✘ Pulse pressure may be narrowed, but this is an unreliable sign
E ✘ An ejection systolic murmur is often heard but may be relatively modest in the presence of severe stenosis limiting cardiac output

1.12 A ✘
B ✘ The re-enterant pathway makes atrial dysrhythmias more likely
C ✘ May provoke atrial or ventricular dysrhythmias
D ✔ Associated with long QT syndrome and ventricular dysrhythmias
E ✘ May cause any type of rhythm disturbance

1.13 A ✗ Helpful in both long QT syndromes and vasovagal
syncope
B ✗ Hypokalaemia and diuretic use are associated
C ✔ Romano–Ward syndrome with prolonged QT and
ventricular arrhythmias transmitted as an autosomal
dominant trait
D ✗ Milroy's syndrome, an inherited lymphatic abnormality
E ✗ Resting bradycardia

1.14 A ✗ Due to pulmonary hypertension
B ✔ The left ventricle is usually normal unless there is also MR
C ✗
D ✗ Due to pulmonary hypertension
E ✗ As the stenosis worsens the intensity of the murmur
declines

1.15 A ✗ His risk of a coronary heart disease event in the next
10 years is 43%, although all the measures will help
reduce this risk, the greatest impact will come from
smoking cessation
B ✗
C ✔
D ✗
E ✗

1.16 A ✗ Strongly suggests VT
B ✔ Positive concordance (all chest leads looking similar on
ECG) is found only in patients with ventricular tachycardia
C ✗
D ✗ A rare but useful sign suggesting a ventricular origin
E ✗

1.17 A ✗ Associated with an increased afterload
B ✗
C ✗ Typically causes diastolic LV dysfunction
D ✔ Impairs systolic function – a dilated cardiomyopathy
E ✗

1.18 A ✗
B ✗ As can several other metabolic disorders
C ✗ A Turner's-like syndrome
D ✗ A glycogen storage disorder
E ✔ Neuromyelitis optica, a variant of multiple sclerosis

1.19 A ✗ Over 80% of subjects have minimal symptoms
B ✗ Tachycardia is common in the acute stage
C ✗ ST segment elevation and/or T wave inversion are
common
D ✔ Common
E ✗ But serum troponins are often raised in the acute phase

1.20 A ✗ Typical with moderate left-to-right shunt volume
     B ✔ A feature of a 'benign venous hum' in children
     C ✗
     D ✗ May occur with right- to-left shunt
     E ✗ Due to increased flow across the mitral valve

1.21 A ✗ Reversed splitting suggests impaired conduction
     B ✔ Typical finding in left bundle branch block
     C ✗ Conduction abnormalities are likely
     D ✗ Left ventricular outflow obstruction
     E ✗ Left ventricular outflow obstruction

1.22 A ✗ Male:female ratio is 1.5:1
     B ✗
     C ✗ A principal sign
     D ✗ But more common in the coronaries
     E ✔ As are changes in the lips, hands, tongue, and conjunctivae

1.23 A ✗ Autosomal dominant with 50% chance of inheriting the trait
     B ✗ Consist primarily of triglycerides
     C ✗ The nephrotic syndrome increases plasma cholesterol and triglycerides
     D ✔ But does not prolong life
     E ✗ Increases progressively with age

1.24 A ✔ In 50% of cases of endocarditis, the organism arises from the oropharynx
     B ✗ Not bactericidal; benzylpenicillin and amoxicillin should be used
     C ✗ Renal failure reverses with treatment of endocarditis
     D ✗ Valve replacement is indicated at all stages of treatment if LVF develops
     E ✗ Timing blood cultures with peaks of pyrexia does not increase the yield of positive cultures; six to eight samples should be taken in the first 24 hours

1.25 A ✗ 'CV' waves due to rise in right atrial pressure during ventricular systole
     B ✗ Usually a loud P_2 signifying pulmonary hypertension
     C ✔ Secondary to pulmonary hypertension
     D ✗
     E ✗ Characteristically increases with inspiration

1.26 A ✗ Coarctation is likely to be just distal to the left subclavian artery
     B ✗ Incidence of aortic stenosis and aortic dissection is increased
     C ✗ But also causes aortic dissection
     D ✗ Coarctation produces a systolic murmur only
     E ✔ due to hypertension, atheroma, dissection and berry aneurysms

1.27 A ✔ Also seen in hypercalcaemia
B ✘ Clockwise rotation
C ✘ A late sign of acute infarction, ST elevation is usually seen first
D ✘ The normal QT is less than 440 msec and is rate dependent
E ✘ Mobitz type I (Wenckebach) block has a lengthening of the PR interval; Mobitz type II has a fixed PR interval

1.28 A ✘
B ✔ Unlike ventricular fibrillation within the first 12 hours
C ✘ Indicates acceptable LV function
D ✘ But coexisting diseases are more common, e.g. diabetes
E ✘ Inferior infarcts tend to cause less damage and have a better prognosis

1.29 A ✘ Can reveal left atrial enlargement but not accurately quantify the size: echocardiography is much better
B ✘ Typically normal, the right ventricle lies within the cardiac silhouette
C ✘ Typically decreased CT ratio
D ✘ Good correlation but better with the ECG and echocardiogram
E ✔ And can be confusing

1.30 A ✘ Gradients greater than 50 mmHg
B ✘ Pulmonary artery oxygen saturation reflects cardiac output as the arteriovenous oxygen saturation difference increases as cardiac output falls
C ✘ 0.2% mortality
D ✘
E ✔

1.31 A ✔ Accessory pathway of Kent
B ✘ Atrial pacing can control atrial tachycardias
C ✘ AF occurs in about 15% of patients
D ✘ Possibly as a result of atrial natriuretic peptide release
E ✘ Impossible to distinguish from the severity of patient distress

1.32 A ✘ Mitral incompetence due to a prolapsing mitral valve
B ✘ Suggests a pulmonary flow murmur
C ✘ Radionuclide ventriculography or angiography
D ✘ Loud third HS due to rapid ventricular filling in early diastole
E ✔ Common and rarely troublesome

1.33 A ✘ Right-to-left
B ✘
C ✘ The 'jet lesion' occurs on the right ventricle
D ✘ Localized to the left sternal edge and associated with a palpable thrill
E ✔

1.34 A ✗ Usually associated with aortic incompetence
     B ✗ Usually maximal from the onset
     C ✗ Typically a tachycardia
     D ✗ Most patients have had longstanding hypertension
     E ✔ Due to leak, reaction or underlying aortic inflammation

1.35 A ✗ Characteristically within the previous 3–4 weeks
     B ✗ Indicates mitral valvitis
     C ✗ Unlike SLE or adult Still's disease
     D ✗
     E ✔ Usually an additive, pauciarticular, large joint arthropathy

1.36 A ✗ Typically causes a congestive cardiomyopathy
     B ✗
     C ✗ CCF occurs in 10%
     D ✔ Also haemochromatosis
     E ✗

1.37 A ✗ Hypoxia causes pulmonary vasoconstriction and
          hypertension
     B ✗
     C ✗ Increased vascular resistance
     D ✗
     E ✔

1.38 A ✗
     B ✔ PCI would be too hazardous
     C ✗ Anti-anginal therapy alleviates symptoms
     D ✗ High risk from surgery
     E ✗ Risk of surgery is greater than the risk from variant angina

1.39 A ✗
     B ✗ A rare diagnosis
     C ✔ Pseudo-Cushing's syndrome associated with alcohol use
     D ✗
     E ✗

1.40 A ✗ Patients with prosthetic valves are particularly vulnerable
          to endocarditis
     B ✗
     C ✔ For prosthetic valves with a tilting disc or a ball
     D ✗ Indicates thrombus developing at the valve
     E ✗ Interaction with warfarin enhances the anticoagulant effect

Clinical sciences and statistics

QUESTIONS

2.1 In a phase II trial of a new drug, 20 out of 100 people treated with the active drug died compared with 25 out of 100 people given the placebo. Which ONE of the following statements is TRUE?
A The relative risk reduction is 5%
B The number needed to treat to prevent 1 death is 20
C An analysis of variance (ANOVA) is the most appropriate statistical test to apply to the data
D Randomization for entry to the study is always required
E Student's t-test would be an appropriate statistical tool to assess significance

2.2 A scientist wishes to compare serum asymmetric dimethylarginine levels, an inhibitor of nitric oxide production, in two distinct groups. Within each group, the range of plasma levels exhibits a skewed rather than a normal distribution. Which ONE of the following statistical tests would be the most appropriate to assess differences between the serum levels within the two groups?
A Paired Student's t-test
B Wilcoxon rank sum test
C Spearman's rank correlation
D Chi-squared test
E Bonferroni's test

2.3 Which ONE of the following statistical processes is LEAST likely to reduce the possibility of systematic errors arising from a clinical study?
A Logarithmic transformation
B Stratification
C Randomization
D Restricted entry criteria
E Logistic regression

2.4 **A drug company wishes to conduct a randomized, placebo-controlled study to investigate the effect of a novel drug on the frequency of hospital admissions in patients with asthma. Which ONE of the following factors will NOT affect the sample size required for the study?**

A The anticipated rate of hospital admission in the control group

B The difference in admission rates between the two groups

C The desired level of statistical significance

D Drug tolerability

E The choice of post-hoc statistical analysis

2.5 **Which ONE of the following statements best describes the arithmetic mean of a series of measurements?**

A The most commonly occurring value

B The value intermediate between the highest and lowest measurement

C Twice the median

D The average value of all the measurements

E The sum of values of measurement multiplied by the number of measurements

2.6 **Which ONE of the following statements about normally distributed data is TRUE?**

A The data are likely to exhibit considerable skew of the values about the mean

B The mode and median coincide with the mean

C 95% of the area under the curve is represented by the mean plus or minus one standard deviation

D The standard error of the mean is the standard deviation of the mean multiplied by the square of the number of observations (N)

E All people in the sample are normal

2.7 **Which ONE of the following statements about the Student's t-test is FALSE?**

A It was developed specifically for use by students

B It cannot be used to compare two normally distributed samples

C It requires reference tables for statistical assessment of the 't' value

D It does not require calculation of the standard error of the differences between two medians

E It uses the concepts of degrees of freedom and confidence limits

2.8 Which ONE of the following statements about the chi-square test is TRUE?
A The test makes comparisons between groups
B The test is more useful if small numbers are present
C The test requires prior calculation of the potency ratio
D A probability $P < 0.1$ indicates statistical significance
E The test compares actual values rather than proportions or number of occurrences

2.9 Which ONE of the following statements about the incidence of a disease is TRUE?
A It is the number of cases of disease present at any given time in the sample under study
B It is a measure of only clinical rather than subclinical cases
C The incidence of a chronic disease is typically less than its prevalence
D It is a useful measure in determining the cause of a disease
E It is best determined from post-mortem data

2.10 Which ONE of the following statements about the transmitter nitric oxide is TRUE?
A It is synthesized from L-citrulline
B It is a potent vasoconstrictor
C It increases plasma cyclic AMP
D It is stored in vesicles for release
E It is soluble in blood

2.11 Which ONE of the following statements about atrial natriuretic peptide is TRUE?
A It is secreted mainly by the kidney
B It increases the production and release of renin
C Cyclic GMP is the main second messenger in signal transduction
D It increases blood pressure
E It induces vasopressin secretion by the posterior pituitary

2.12 Which ONE of the following statements about the neuronal action potential is TRUE?
A Myelination decreases nerve conduction velocity
B Large fibres conduct more slowly than small fibres
C Inactivation of potassium channels causes the refractory period
D Tetrodotoxin blocks voltage gated sodium channels
E Depolarization results from inhibition of sodium entry during potassium efflux

2.13   A 54-year-old man is admitted semi-conscious with a normal blood pressure but evidence of peripheral cyanosis. Urinalysis showed no evidence of ketonuria and arterial blood gases showed a pH 6.9, $PaCO_2$ 2.0 KPa, PaO_2 12.7 KPa, HCO_3^- 3.0 mmol/L. Blood glucose was 6.1 mmol/L and the anion gap was 28 mmol/L with a plasma lactate 17.0 mmol/L. Which ONE of the following diagnoses is most consistent with these findings?

A   Diabetic ketoacidosis
B   Ingestion of excess ammonium chloride
C   Chronic renal failure
D   Ingestion of ethylene glycol
E   Primary hyperaldosteronism

2.14   Which ONE of the following statements about prostacyclin (PGI2) is TRUE?

A   It is synthesized by smooth muscle cells
B   It is formed from arachidonic acid by the action of lipoxygenase
C   It is a potent vasoconstrictor
D   It inhibits platelet aggregation
E   It causes uterine contraction in the non-pregnant state

2.15   Which ONE of the following sugars is a monosaccharide?

A   Galactose
B   Lactose
C   Sucrose
D   Maltose
E   Starch

2.16   In which ONE of the following genetic disorders is the metabolism of amino acids normal?

A   Phenylketonuria
B   Albinism
C   Gaucher's disease
D   Homocystinuria
E   Maple syrup urine disease

2.17   Which ONE of the following statements about haemoglobin is TRUE?

A   Each haemoglobin molecule comprises two haem groups
B   Each haem group binds four molecules of oxygen
C   Within the haem group, iron is in the ferric state (Fe^{3+})
D   Globin consists of two polypeptide chains
E   Haemoglobin A_2 contains both alpha and delta chains

2.18   Which ONE of the following factors is likely to shift the oxygen dissociation curve to the right?

A   Methaemoglobinaemia
B   Alkalosis
C   Decreased blood 2,3 diphosphoglycerate levels
D   A fall in body temperature
E   Decreased arterial partial pressure of carbon dioxide

2.19 **Which ONE of the following metabolic actions is associated with adrenaline (epinephrine)?**
A   Glyconeogenesis
B   Decreased fatty acid utilization by muscle
C   Decreased lipolysis in adipocytes
D   Decreased ketone body production by the liver
E   Inhibition of adenyl cyclase via alpha-adrenergic receptors

2.20 **Which ONE of the following statements about vitamin deficiency states is TRUE?**
A   Riboflavin deficiency causes dryness of the mouth and genitalia
B   Pyridoxine deficiency causes proximal myopathy
C   Vitamin A deficiency causes exfoliative dermatitis
D   Niacin deficiency causes congestive cardiomyopathy
E   Folic acid deficiency causes glossitis but not stomatitis

2.21 **Which ONE of the following statements about the enzyme guanyly cyclase is TRUE?**
A   The enzyme is inhibited by isosorbide mononitrate
B   It inhibits the effect of natriuretic peptides
C   It catalyses the formation of cyclic GMP from GTP
D   Its activity is enhanced by phosphodiesterases
E   The enzyme contains a haem group which binds nitric oxide

2.22 **Which part of the renal medulla is responsible for the majority of renal tubular reabsorption of bicarbonate in normal physiological states?**
A   Distal convoluted tubules
B   Thick ascending loop of Henle
C   Collecting ducts
D   Proximal convoluted tubules
E   Inner medullary collecting ducts

2.23 **Which ONE of the following statements about the cranial foramina is TRUE?**
A   The jugular foramen contains the cranial nerve XII
B   The hypoglossal foramen contains the cranial nerve X
C   The stylomastoid foramen contains the cranial nerve V
D   The foramen lacerum contains the internal carotid artery
E   The foramen magnum contains the cranial nerve VIII

2.24 **Which ONE of the following actions is mediated by beta-2 adrenergic receptors?**
A   Bronchoconstriction
B   Vasoconstriction
C   Uterine contraction
D   Decreased sweat gland secretion
E   Insulin secretion

2.25 **Which ONE of the following muscles is innervated by the median nerve?**
A   Extensor pollicis longus
B   Flexor carpi ulnaris
C   Abductor pollicis
D   The medial two lumbricals
E   Extensor pollicis brevis

2.26 **Which ONE of the following ions is present in higher concentrations in the intracellular fluid compartment than the extracellular fluid compartment?**
A   Sodium
B   Magnesium
C   Chloride
D   Bicarbonate
E   Calcium

2.27 **A 47-year-old woman complains of the recent onset of shortness of breath. The past medical history included lung surgery for an unexplained mass on the chest X-ray which later proved to be a benign tumour. Isotope lung scanning revealed a low ventilation to perfusion (V/Q) ratio. Which ONE of the following disorders would best explain these findings?**
A   A right-to-left shunt of blood
B   Pneumothorax
C   Surgical removal of a lung
D   Lobar pneumonia
E   Fibrosing alveolitis

2.28 **Which ONE of the following conditions is associated with increased gastric motility?**
A   Anorexia nervosa
B   Gastrinoma
C   Vestibular neuronitis
D   Acute intermittent porphyria
E   Partial gastrectomy

2.29 **Which ONE of the following gastrointestinal neuropeptides increases colonic motility?**
A   Peptide YY
B   Enteroglucagon
C   Calcitonin gene-related peptide
D   Somatostatin
E   Neurotensin

2.30 **In which ONE of the following disorders is autosomal dominant inheritance the most common mode of inheritance?**
A   Gilbert's syndrome
B   Limb girdle muscular dystrophy
C   Cystic fibrosis
D   Spinal muscular atrophy
E   Beta-thalassaemia

2.31 In which ONE of the following disorders is autosomal recessive inheritance the most common mode of inheritance?
A   Hereditary haemorrhagic telangiectasia
B   Hereditary spherocytosis
C   Wilson's disease
D   Familial hypercholesterolaemia
E   Pseudohypoparathyroidism

2.32 The family history suggests an X-linked recessive disorder. Which ONE of the following statements is TRUE?
A   Half of the sons of a female carrier are carriers
B   Half of the daughters of affected males are carriers
C   All of the sons of an affected male are normal
D   There is a 1 in 2 chance of a child of a female carrier being affected
E   Heterozygous females are likely to be affected by the disorder

2.33 Which ONE of the following statements about acetyl coenzyme A is TRUE?
A   It is converted into formic acid in the tricarboxylic acid cycle (Kreb's cycle)
B   Its production from pyruvate is controlled by positive feedback
C   It inhibits glucose-6-phosphate production from fructose-6-phosphate in the cell
D   Conversion to fatty acids is an energy-consuming action
E   Its production from citrate is the result of oxidative phosphorylation

2.34 Which ONE of the following is the MAJOR constituent of very-low-density lipoprotein (VLDL)?
A   Triacylglyceride
B   Apolipoprotein A-II
C   Cholesterol
D   Phospholipid
E   Protein

2.35 Which ONE of the following tests is based on an immunofluorescent technique?
A   Factor VIII assay in haemophilia
B   The Rose–Waaler test in rheumatoid arthritis
C   The TPHA test in syphilis
D   Identification of tumour-specific antigens in sera
E   Detection of tissue immunoglobulins

2.36 Which ONE of the following statements about immunoglobulins is TRUE?
A   They are secreted by transformed T lymphocytes
B   The lamina propria of the gut produces predominantly IgG
C   IgM and IgA cross the placenta
D   IgD is found on the surface of immature B lymphocytes
E   IgE is predominantly involved in immune complex formation

2.37   **Which ONE of the following statements about the complement system is TRUE?**
A   Only the classical pathway produces both C3 and C5 convertase
B   Components of the classical pathway are mainly beta-globulins
C   The classical pathway is triggered by bacterial endotoxin
D   The alternative pathway is triggered by platelet aggregation
E   C1 esterase excess produces angio-oedema

2.38   **Which ONE of the following is an expected physiological change associated with the normal ageing process?**
A   Decreased calcium phosphate content per 100 g bone
B   Increased tissue sensitivity to insulin
C   Reduced numbers of pacing cells within the sino-atrial node
D   Increased glomerular filtration rate
E   Increased suppressor T cell function

2.39   **Which ONE of the following factors in healthy elderly individuals is MOST responsible for the increase in susceptibility to hypothermia?**
A   An increased core-skin temperature gradient
B   Increased ability to detect small changes in room temperature
C   An impaired ability to shiver effectively in response to cooling
D   Impaired cellular responses to thyroid hormones
E   Thermoregulation which is not altered by autonomic function

2.40   **Which ONE of the following factors is MOST responsible for the increased risk of falls in elderly subjects compared with younger individuals?**
A   A reduced variability of step length
B   An increased step frequency
C   An increased step width
D   An increased step length
E   A reduced antero-posterior sway in women than men

2.41   **Which ONE of the following statements about haemophilia A is TRUE?**
A   Half of the sons of a female carrier are carriers
B   All daughters of an affected male will be carriers
C   All sons of an affected male will be carriers
D   1 in 2 of all the children of a female carrier will be affected
E   Homozygous females are unaffected

2.42   **Which ONE of the following statements about the human genome is TRUE?**
A   Somatic cell nuclei contain 23 pairs of homologous autosomes
B   Gamete nuclei are diploid with a single X or Y chromosome
C   The X chromosome is smaller than the Y chromosome
D   An F body in somatic cell nuclei represents a Y chromosome
E   A Barr body is a genetically inactive X chromosome

2.43 Which ONE of the following cellular events occurs in the cytoplasm rather than within the cell nucleus?
A Transcription to mRNA precursor
B DNA replication
C Translation of mRNA to gene product
D Excision of introns and splicing of exons
E Control of gene expression

2.44 Which ONE of the following is an essential amino acid?
A Leucine
B Glycine
C Hydroxylysine
D Arginine
E Glutamine

2.45 Which ONE of the following cell receptors activates adenylate cyclase?
A Insulin
B Alpha-2 adrenoceptor
C Histamine 1
D Thromboxane A2
E Thyroid-stimulating hormone

2.46 Which ONE of the following tumours is associated with the proto-oncogene c-*myc*?
A Colon carcinoma
B Breast carcinoma
C Cervical carcinoma
D Small-cell lung carcinoma
E Burkitt's lymphoma

2.47 Which ONE of the following statements about the release of free fatty acid from adipose tissue is TRUE?
A It is increased by noradrenaline (norepinephrine)
B It is increased by insulin
C It is decreased by glucocorticoids
D It is decreased by growth hormone
E It is dependent on activated pancreatic lipase

2.48 Which ONE of the following statements about normal cerebrospinal fluid is TRUE?
A CSF is under less hydrostatic pressure than the venous sinuses of brain
B CSF is present within the subdural space
C Lateral ventricles communicate with the third ventricle via the foramen of Munro
D The total CSF volume is approximately 500 ml
E CSF is produced by the arachnoid villi

2.49   A 29-year-old man is admitted with a fever without localizing signs. Blood cultures yield a Gram-negative diplococcus. Which ONE of the following is the likeliest infecting organism?

A   *Neisseria meningitidis*
B   *Streptococcus pneumoniae*
C   *Corynebacterium diphtheria*
D   *Staphylococcus aureus*
E   *Borrelia burgdorferi*

2.50   Which ONE of the following statements about the spinal cord is TRUE?

A   The dorsal columns predominantly convey pain and temperature sensation
B   Spinothalamic fibres from the sacral segments lie innermost
C   The cauda equina begins at the level of the first sacral vertebra
D   The anterior spinal artery supplies the sensory compartments
E   The dorsal root ganglion lies within the subarachnoid space

ANSWERS

2.1 A ✗ The absolute risk reduction is 5% and relative risk reduction is 20%

B ✔ The number needed to treat = 1/absolute risk reduction 1/0.05 (i.e. 5%) = 20

C ✗

D ✗

E ✗ Used for test values that are normally distributed

2.2 A ✗ The data are not normally distributed so a non-parametric test is indicated. Paired t-tests are not appropriate for unrelated samples

B ✔ Non-parametric test; Mann–Whitney U test can also be used

C ✗ Useful when observations are difficult to quantify

D ✗ Useful for analysing data grouped by category, e.g. eye colour

E ✗ A 'correction' that is used when making multiple comparisons, to reduce the likelihood of false positive results.

2.3 A ✔ Used to compare data sets that have different variances or are non-normally distributed

B ✗

C ✗ All reduce selection bias to reduce sampling errors, i.e. biases in the data

D ✗

E ✗

2.4 A ✗

B ✗ The power of the study depends on the sample size, frequency of the main outcome measure, size of effect one wishes to detect, and the significance level desired

C ✗

D ✗ If patients drop out because of drug intolerance, this will reduce drug efficacy and reduce the power of the study. An allowance for drop-outs is necessary in calculating the sample size required

E ✔ By definition these are tests done in addition to the primary analysis and should not influence the sample size calculation

---

2.5 A ✗ This is the mode

B ✗

C ✗

D ✔

E ✗

2.6   A   ✗   Non-skewed or parametric data
     B   ✔   The mode is the value that occurs most frequently; the median is the middle value
     C   ✗   95% is mean plus or minus <u>two</u> standard deviations
     D   ✗   Standard deviation of the mean divided by the square root of N
     E   ✗

2.7   A   ✗   Pseudonym of the mathematician, William Gosset
     B   ✗
     C   ✗
     D   ✗   means not medians
     E   ✔   95% confidence limits = (1.96 × standard error) < and > the mean

2.8   A   ✔   The null hypothesis that there is no difference between groups is being tested
     B   ✗   Often Yates correction required if numbers < 40 and this reduces value of chi-square
     C   ✗
     D   ✗   Any chance less than 1 in 20 ($P < 0.05$)
     E   ✗   The test is designed to compare proportions rather than actual values, e.g. the number of patients losing weight, not their mean weight loss

2.9   A   ✗   This is the prevalence of a disease (includes all cases)
     B   ✗
     C   ✔   Less than the prevalence; the incidence is the number of new cases arising each year
     D   ✗
     E   ✗

2.10 A   ✗   L-arginine is the substrate producing nitric oxide and L-citrulline
     B   ✗   A vasodilator in systemic and pulmonary circulations
     C   ✗   Increases cGMP
     D   ✗   Too highly reactive to be stored
     E   ✔   Highly soluble due to its high affinity for haemoglobin

2.11 A   ✗   It is synthesized and released by atrial myocytes in response to the stimulus of atrial stretch
     B   ✗   It inhibits renin production
     C   ✔   Catalysed by guanylyl cyclase
     D   ✗   It is a vasodilator and lowers blood pressure
     E   ✗   It inhibits vasopressin secretion

2.12 A   ✗   Myelination increases the conduction velocity
     B   ✗   Small fibres conduct more slowly than large ones
     C   ✗   Due to inactivation of voltage-gated sodium channels
     D   ✔   Tetrodotoxin is produced by the puffer or blow fish
     E   ✗   Repolarization results from the inhibition of sodium entry

2.13 A ✗ Normal blood glucose; peripheral perfusion is common in severe acidosis including diabetic ketoacidosis
B ✗ Causes metabolic alkalosis with a normal anion gap
C ✗ Unusual to get such severe lactic acidosis
D ✔ May occur with aspirin (but respiratory alkalosis is more typical)
E ✗ Alkalosis is characteristic

2.14 A ✗ It is synthesized in endothelial cells and <u>acts</u> on smooth muscle cells
B ✗ It is formed by the action of cyclo-oxygenase on arachidonic acid
C ✗ Vasodilator lowering both systemic and pulmonary vascular resistance
D ✔
E ✗ PGE inhibits contractility of the non-pregnant uterus but stimulates the pregnant uterus

2.15 A ✔ Also glucose and fructose
B ✗ Glucose and galactose
C ✗
D ✗ Glucose dimer
E ✗ Maltose polymer

2.16 A ✗ Error in converting phenylalanine to tyrosine (phenylalanine hydroxylase deficiency)
B ✗ Error in tyrosinase pathway (tyrosinase deficiency)
C ✔ Defective alpha-glucosidase affecting sphingolipid metabolism
D ✗ Defective cystathione beta-synthase
E ✗ Defective branched chain keto-acid decarboxylase

2.17 A ✗ Each comprises four haem groups
B ✗ Each haem group binds one oxygen molecule
C ✗ The ferrous state (Fe^{2+}); Fe^{3+} occurs in methaemoglobinaemia
D ✗ Contains four polypeptide chains
E ✔ HbA_2 comprises two alpha and two delta chains

2.18 A ✔ Carboxyhaemoglobin shifts the curve to the left
B ✗ The effect of pH on the ODC is called the Bohr effect
C ✗ 2,3 DPG lowers affinity of haemoglobin for O_2
D ✗
E ✗

2.19 A ✗ Adrenaline (epinephrine) like glucagon promotes glycogenolysis
B ✗ Increased muscle fatty acid utilization
C ✗ Increases fatty acid release from adipocytes
D ✗ Increased hepatic ketone body production
E ✔ Unlike the beta receptors which activate adenyl cyclase

2.20   A   ✔   And cracking of the skin around the mouth, ears and eyelids
      B   ✘   Peripheral neuropathy
      C   ✘   Causes xerophthalmia, especially if complicated by measles
      D   ✘   Niacin deficiency causes pellagra (dermatitis, diarrhoea and dementia)
      E   ✘   Causes both associated with megaloblastic anaemia

2.21   A   ✘   Stimulated by nitrates, an effect mediated by nitric oxide
      B   ✘   ANP and BNP both increase cyclic GMP levels
      C   ✔
      D   ✘   Phosphodiesterases mediate the degradation of cGMP
      E   ✘   The NO-haem complex changes the molecule's shape resulting in a 200-fold increase in the catalytic effects of the enzyme

2.22   A   ✘   <5%
      B   ✘   15%
      C   ✘   <5%
      D   ✔   75%
      E   ✘   Negligible

2.23   A   ✘   Cranial nerve X
      B   ✘   Cranial nerve XII
      C   ✘   Cranial nerve V exits via the foramen rotundum and ovale
      D   ✔
      E   ✘   The foramen magnum contains the cranial nerve XI

2.24   A   ✘   Bronchodilatation
      B   ✘   Vasodilatation
      C   ✘   Uterine relaxation in the pregnant state
      D   ✘   Increased sweat gland secretion
      E   ✔

2.25   A   ✘   Supplied by the radial nerve
      B   ✘   Supplied by the ulnar nerve
      C   ✔   Also the opponens pollicis
      D   ✘   Only the lateral two lumbricals
      E   ✘   Supplied by the radial nerve

2.26   A   ✘
      B   ✔   40 times greater in the intracellular compartment
      C   ✘
      D   ✘
      E   ✘   Similar concentrations in intra- and extracellular fluid

2.27   A   ✔   Non-perfused lung
      B   ✘   High V/Q ratio
      C   ✘   No change overall in the V/Q ratio
      D   ✘   High V/Q ratio
      E   ✘   High V/Q ratio

2.28	A	✗	Reduces gastric emptying
	B	✔	
	C	✗	Decreases motility due to labyrinthine stimulation
	D	✗	Decreases motility
	E	✗	

2.29	A	✗	Co-localized with enteroglucagon — 'ileal + colonic brake'
	B	✗	Released from L cells in the distal ileum; reduces motility
	C	✗	CGRP stimulates the release of VIP, decreasing motility
	D	✗	Decreases motility and inhibits secretion
	E	✔	Released from N cells in the distal ileum

2.30	A	✔	
	B	✗	Autosomal recessive
	C	✗	Autosomal recessive
	D	✗	Autosomal recessive
	E	✗	Autosomal recessive

2.31	A	✗	Autosomal dominant (Rendu–Osler–Weber syndrome)
	B	✗	Usually autosomal dominant affecting 1–2 per 10 000
	C	✔	Chromosome 13 defect causing hepato-lenticular degeneration
	D	✗	Autosomal dominant
	E	✗	X-linked dominant mode of inheritance predominates

2.32	A	✗	50% of daughters are carriers. 50% of sons are affected
	B	✗	All daughters of affected males are carriers
	C	✔	Because only the X chromosome is passed to daughters
	D	✗	1 in 4; 1 in 2 chance of being male; 1 in 2 chance of a male being affected
	E	✗	Only usually affected in the homozygous state

2.33	A	✗	Acetyl CoA is the starting point of Kreb's energy-producing cycle with the production of oxaloacetate
	B	✗	Negative feedback
	C	✗	Glucose-6-phosphate and fructose-6-phosphate are freely convertible but acetyl CoA promotes glucose-6-phosphate and hence glycolysis
	D	✔	Unlike the Kreb's cycle which is energy-producing
	E	✗	Acetyl CoA is formed from the oxidative decarboxylation of <u>pyruvate</u>

2.34	A	✔	About 60% of VLDL
	B	✗	This is a constituent of HDL
	C	✗	About 5% of VLDL
	D	✗	About 14% of VLDL
	E	✗	About 7%

2.35	A	✗	Immunofluorescence is a technique for assessing
	B	✗	cell and tissue structures to identify and
	C	✗	localize particulate proteins such as
	D	✗	immunoglobulins
	E	✔	

37

2.36 A ✗ Secreted by transformed B lymphocytes
 B ✗ IgA; also produced in respiratory tract
 C ✗ IgG is the only immunoglobulin which crosses the placenta
 D ✔
 E ✗ Involved in hypersensitivity reactions

2.37 A ✗ Both classical and alternative pathways produce C3 convertase
 B ✔ Synthesized in liver
 C ✗ } Alternative pathway; the classical pathway is
 D ✗ } triggered when immune complex combines with C1q
 E ✗ C1q esterase deficiency produces congenital angio-oedema

2.38 A ✗ Bone mass declines (osteoporosis) but mineralization is normal
 B ✗ Reduced insulin sensitivity and glucose tolerance declines
 C ✔ Limits ability to mount a tachycardia
 D ✗ Decreased number of nephrons, GFR and medullary function
 E ✗ Decreased function may contribute to increase in autoimmune disease

2.39 A ✗ Decreased below normal (normal value 4°C)
 B ✗ Elderly can detect changes > 2°C cf 1°C change in younger people
 C ✔ Metabolic heat production is 50% < than younger people
 D ✗ Thyroid function is normal
 E ✗ Autonomic dysfunction impairs thermoregulation especially in the elderly

2.40 A ✗ Increased step length variability
 B ✗ Decreased step frequency and a slower gait
 C ✔ A broader-based gait
 D ✗ Shorter steps
 E ✗ A-P sway is greater in females than men in all the adult age groups

2.41 A ✗ X-linked recessive; 50% daughters are carriers, 50% sons are affected
 B ✔
 C ✗ Remember only the X chromosome passes from father to daughters
 D ✗ 1 in 4 chance of being affected
 E ✗ Homozygosity in females

2.42 A ✗ 22 pairs plus two sex chromosomes
 B ✗ Gamete nuclei are haploid
 C ✗ The Y chromosome is the smaller
 D ✗ Fluorescent spots on interphase nuclei of male cells
 E ✔

2.43 A ✗ Direct copying of one strand of DNA occurs in all nuclei
     B ✗
     C ✔ A cytoplasmic event
     D ✗ Forms the processed mRNA
     E ✗

2.44 A ✔⎫ The eight essential amino acids are
     B ✗ ⎬ methionine, lysine, tryptophan, phenylalanine,
     C ✗ ⎭ leucine, isoleucine, threonine and valine
     D ✗
     E ✗

2.45 A ✗ Intrinsic protein tyrosine kinase activity
     B ✗ Inhibits adenylate cyclase
     C ✗⎱ Histamine 2 and prostacyclin
     D ✗⎰ activate adenylate cyclase
     E ✔

2.46 A ✔ C-*ras*
     B ✗
     C ✗
     D ✗
     E ✗

2.47 A ✔ Rapidly as happens in fear or cold
     B ✗ Decreased rapidly as blood glucose rises
     C ✗ Increased slowly, in response to stress
     D ✗ Increased slowly, in response to hunger
     E ✗ Dependent on activated lipoprotein lipase

2.48 A ✗ Greater
     B ✗ Subarachnoid space
     C ✔
     D ✗ Total volume 120–150 ml
     E ✗ Produced by the choroid plexuses; arachnoid villi reabsorb
         CSF

2.49 A ✔
     B ✗ Gram-positive coccus
     C ✗ Gram-positive aerobic
     D ✗ Gram-positive coccus
     E ✗ Flagellated spirochaete

2.50 A ✗ Vibration and proprioception
     B ✗
     C ✗ Spinal cord ends at the first lumbar vertebra
     D ✗ Supplies principally the anterior (motor) components
     E ✔

3

Clinical pharmacology, therapeutics and toxicology

QUESTIONS

3.1 A 34-year-old woman has been taking lithium for 10 years as a treatment for mania. Her plasma levels have always been in the therapeutic range. Which ONE of the following is LEAST LIKELY to be attributable to lithium toxicity?
A   Tremor
B   Hypothyroidism
C   Hyponatraemia
D   Rhabdomyolysis
E   Weight gain

3.2 Which ONE of the following antagonists is MOST LIKELY to show non-competitive antagonistic properties at therapeutic doses?
A   Ketamine
B   Lisinopril
C   Aspirin
D   Pindolol
E   Naloxone

3.3 A 64-year-old woman who has recently started several medications subsequently develops epilepsy for the first time. Which ONE of the following drugs is LEAST LIKELY to be responsible for her seizures?
A   Ciprofloxacin
B   Aminophylline
C   Phenytoin
D   Captopril
E   Prochlorperazine

3.4 Which ONE of the following phenomena is LEAST likely to be attributable to reversible competitive antagonism?
A   A shift in the dose response curve to the right
B   A linear increase in the dose ratio with increasing antagonist concentrations
C   Exhibition of surmountability
D   Non-covalent binding of a drug with its receptor
E   An alteration in the affinity of the agonist for the receptor

3.5   Which ONE of the following statements about the dose response relationship of drugs acting on only one type of receptor is TRUE?
   A   It is most likely to be linear
   B   It can be used to calculate the equilibrium dissociation constant (Kd)
   C   Addition of an irreversible antagonist will not alter the maximum response obtained
   D   Partial agonists are unable to produce a maximal response
   E   Differences in potency between drugs are manifested by variation in the maximum response obtained

3.6   In which ONE of the following drug overdoses is haemodialysis LEAST likely to be clinically useful in the management of severe poisoning?
   A   Methanol
   B   Salicylates
   C   Iron
   D   Lithium
   E   Phenobarbitone

3.7   For patients on long-term therapy, in which ONE of the following drug therapies is therapeutic drug monitoring LEAST LIKELY to be clinically useful?
   A   Phenytoin
   B   Ciclosporin
   C   Sodium valproate
   D   Lithium
   E   Carbamazepine

3.8   A 66-year-old man presents with malaise, cough, increasing shortness of breath and a ground-glass appearance on his chest radiograph. Which ONE of the following drugs is LEAST LIKELY to be responsible?
   A   Captopril
   B   Nitrofurantoin
   C   Methysergide
   D   Bleomycin
   E   Azathioprine

3.9   Which ONE of the following drug therapies is MOST LIKELY to cause a problem for an individual with glucose–6-phosphate dehydrogenase deficiency?
   A   Aspirin
   B   Amoxicillin
   C   Propranolol
   D   Amitriptyline
   E   Trimethoprim

3.10 **Which ONE of the following statements about lipid-lowering drug therapy is TRUE?**
A   Statins increase the activity of HMG CoA reductase
B   Statins increase plasma LDL concentrations
C   Nicotinic acid increases lipolysis and decreases HDL concentrations
D   Fibrates decrease VLDL lipolysis
E   Colestipol decreases intestinal reabsorption of bile acids

3.11 **A 37-year-old woman who is concerned about obesity weighs 90 Kg and has a fasting blood glucose of 9.7 mmol/L. Which ONE of the following drug therapies is MOST likely to promote weight loss rather than weight gain?**
A   Oral contraceptives
B   Pizotifen
C   Amitriptyline
D   Fluoxetine
E   Glipizide

3.12 **A 20-year-old female, who is established on the oral contraceptive pill, is admitted following a second seizure. Laboratory analysis confirms a urinary tract infection. Which ONE of the following agents is LEAST LIKELY to increase the risks of an unwanted pregnancy?**
A   Phenytoin
B   Carbamazepine
C   Sodium valproate
D   Tetracycline
E   Ampicillin

3.13 **A 27-year-old depressed woman presents following a drug overdose with dilated pupils, seizures, tachycardia and a prolonged PR interval on her ECG. Which ONE of the following drugs is the MOST LIKELY cause of the clinical features present?**
A   Phenytoin
B   Theophylline
C   Imipramine
D   Aspirin
E   Iron

3.14 **Which ONE of the following statements about chronic therapy with angiotensin converting enzyme (ACE) inhibitors is TRUE?**
A   Cough occurs in ~25% of individuals
B   Plasma renin activity falls
C   Plasma potassium falls
D   Bradykinin metabolism is impaired
E   First dose hypotension is a particular problem in hypertensive individuals

3.15 Which ONE of the following drugs can safely be given to a woman in the 29th week of pregnancy?
A Captopril
B Warfarin
C Misoprostol
D Tetracycline
E Bendroflumethiazide (bendrofluazide)

3.16 Which ONE of the following statements about drug metabolism in normal pregnancy is TRUE?
A The volume of distribution is likely to decrease
B The plasma concentration of drugs that are highly protein bound is likely to increase
C Renal clearance of drugs excreted by the kidneys is likely to decrease
D Absorption of orally administered drugs is likely to decrease
E Hepatic drug metabolism is likely to increase

3.17 In which ONE of the following drug therapies is the mode of drug metabolism likely to be unaffected by genetic differences in drug metabolism between individuals?
A Captopril
B Isoniazid
C Atenolol
D Succinylcholine
E Proguanil

3.18 A 16-year-old girl is admitted having collapsed at a night club where she is thought to have consumed a tablet of ecstasy (MDMA). Which ONE of the following clinical features suggests an alternative recreational drug has been ingested?
A Tachycardia
B Pin-point pupils
C Hyponatraemia
D Hyperpyrexia
E Metabolic acidosis

3.19 A man is admitted with an acute exacerbation of chronic obstructive pulmonary disease (COPD). Treatment with nebulized salbutamol, steroids, and intravenous aminophylline is commenced. Which ONE of the following drugs started prior to admission is LEAST likely to require an alteration in the dose of aminophylline?
A Ranitidine
B St John's wort
C Ciprofloxacin
D Clarithromycin
E Oral theophylline

3.20 **A drug company wishes to conduct a clinical trial with a novel analgesic agent. Which ONE of the following statements is TRUE?**
A Ethical committee approval is required prior to subject recruitment
B A phase II study typically involves healthy volunteers
C Only serious adverse events need be reported
D A yellow placebo is more likely to be effective than a red one
E Randomization is always required

3.21 **Which ONE of the following statements about drug–enzyme interactions is TRUE?**
A Trihexyphenidyl (benzhexol) increases the activity of acetylcholine esterase
B Lamotrigine inhibits GABA aminotransferase
C Allopurinol inhibits xanthine oxidase
D Carbidopa stimulates the activity of dopamine decarboxylase
E Aspirin activates cyclo-oxygenase

3.22 **Which ONE of the following drugs is correctly paired with an agent which acts as its specific antidote?**
A Diazepam and naloxone
B Ethylene glycol and flumazenil
C Cyanide and methylene blue
D Isoniazid and pyridoxine
E Organophosphate and thioctic acid

3.23 **Which ONE of the following statements about the reporting of adverse drug events in the UK is TRUE?**
A All adverse events should be reported
B Cards should be returned to the Department of Health
C Drugs of particular interest are indicated by a black rectangle in the British National Formulary
D It is not a legal requirement to report adverse reactions
E More than 50% of reactions are reported

3.24 **Which ONE of the following statements about the effects on renal drug excretion by concomitant drug therapy is TRUE?**
A Bendroflumethiazide (bendrofluazide) enhances lithium excretion
B Aspirin increases renal clearance of methotrexate
C Probenecid blocks renal tubular excretion of penicillin
D Ciprofloxacin decreases renal tubular reabsorption of warfarin
E Quinidine enhances the renal clearance of digoxin

3.25 **A 68-year-old man with paroxysmal atrial fibrillation is commenced on amiodarone. Which ONE of the following long-term side-effects is LEAST LIKELY to be attributable to amiodarone?**
A Photosensitivity
B Fibrosing alveolitis
C Hypothyroidism
D Peripheral neuropathy
E Neutropenia

3.26 The following drugs in therapeutic doses exhibit zero-order kinetics (saturable kinetics) with the exception of which ONE drug?

A Phenytoin
B Ethanol
C Fluoxetine
D Nifedipine
E Aspirin

3.27 Which ONE of the following drugs is secreted in human breast milk in concentrations likely to cause a clinically significant risk to the baby?

A Aspirin
B Metformin
C Warfarin
D Mesalazine
E Thyroxine

3.28 Which ONE of the following drugs is LEAST likely to induce bronchospasm in an asthmatic individual?

A Aspirin
B Aminophylline
C Sodium cromoglicate
D Indometacin
E Distigmine bromide

3.29 In which ONE of the following drug therapies is abrupt drug withdrawal following prolonged administration LEAST likely to produce a clinically significant reaction?

A Clonidine
B Corticosteroids
C Propranolol
D Lorazepam
E Warfarin

3.30 Which ONE of the following factors is LEAST likely to affect drug bioavailability?

A Tablet disintegration time
B Gastrointestinal motility
C First-pass hepatic metabolism
D Drug dosage
E Intraluminal gastric pH

3.31 Which ONE of the following drug therapies is LEAST likely to precipitate the onset of malignant hyperthermia in a susceptible individual?

A Decamethonium
B Suxamethonium
C Halothane
D Trichlorethylene
E Dantrolene

3.32 In which ONE of the following drug overdoses is the use of oral therapy with activated charcoal MOST likely to be a useful adjunct in the management of acute poisoning?
A   Boric acid
B   Ferrous sulphate
C   Theophylline
D   Mefenamic acid
E   Lithium carbonate

3.33 Which ONE of the following statements about colchicine therapy is TRUE?
A   It promotes leucocyte migration
B   It is an effective uricosuric drug
C   It is useful in the management of fever of unknown origin
D   It will relieve acute attacks of gout within 12 hours
E   It commonly gives rise to constipation

3.34 A woman with a history of acute intermittent porphyria is admitted with abdominal pain. Which ONE of the following drugs is LEAST likely to precipitate symptoms?
A   Chlorpromazine
B   Oestrogens
C   Griseofulvin
D   Barbiturates
E   Morphine

3.35 A 45-year-old presents with tiredness and is found to have a Coombs-positive haemolytic anaemia. Which ONE of the following drugs is LEAST likely to precipitate haemolysis?
A   Rifampicin
B   Benzylpenicillin
C   Isoniazid
D   Co-trimoxazole
E   Propranolol

3.36 A 24-year-old Indian man is commenced on drug therapy for pulmonary tuberculosis. Which ONE of the following statements about isoniazid therapy is TRUE?
A   It produces a peripheral neuropathy
B   It produces toxic effects more commonly in fast acetylators
C   It is useful as monotherapy for chronic but not acute pulmonary TB
D   It does not cross the blood–brain barrier after oral administration
E   It typically produces a cholestatic jaundice

3.37 **In a symptomatic scrap metal worker, which ONE of the following features is LEAST likely to be attributable to lead poisoning?**
  A Encephalopathy
  B Abdominal colic
  C Macrocytic anaemia
  D Gout
  E Wrist-drop

3.38 **Which ONE of the following statements about intentional drug overdosage is TRUE?**
  A Recent alcohol consumption is often involved
  B A previous history of drug overdosage is unusual
  C Most patients readily admit to suicidal intent
  D Antidepressants are the most commonly taken drug
  E Serious suicidal intent is commoner in females

3.39 **A 15-year-old boy is taken to the casualty department after ingesting approximately 200 ml of aqueous ferrous fumarate 12 hours previously. Which ONE of the following features suggests that an additional poison may also have been consumed?**
  A Burns around the mouth
  B Peripheral cyanosis
  C Haematemesis
  D Drowsiness
  E Metabolic acidosis

3.40 **A 56-year-old man presents with severe polyarticular arthritis. The previous history includes recurrent gout. Which ONE of the following disorders is an absolute contraindication to the use of oral corticosteroid therapy?**
  A Acute gout
  B Systemic hypertension
  C Past history of herpes zoster
  D Herpes simplex keratitis
  E Active duodenal ulceration

3.41 **A 19-year-old student presents acutely unwell to the casualty department, smelling strongly of alcohol. Which ONE of the following features suggests a diagnosis other than that of acute alcoholic intoxication?**
  A Hypoglycaemia
  B Lactic acidosis
  C Hyponatraemia
  D Left ventricular failure
  E Nystagmus, strabismus and unequal pupils

3.42 A known alcoholic is admitted with suspected methyl alcohol (methanol) poisoning. Which ONE of the following statements is TRUE?

A The agent is poorly absorbed from the small bowel
B Toxicity results from the formation of oxaloacetate
C The treatment of choice is ethyl alcohol
D Metabolic alkalosis is a common complication
E Haemodialysis is unlikely to prevent the progression to blindness

3.43 Which ONE of the following cytotoxic agents acts as a pyrimidine antagonist?

A Tioguanine
B Methotrexate
C Vinblastine
D Etoposide
E Cisplatin

3.44 A 34-year-old male farmer presents with collapse following pesticide spraying in a field. Which ONE of the following clinical features cannot be explained by a diagnosis of organophosphorous poisoning?

A Dilated pupils
B Bradycardia
C Hypersalivation
D Pulmonary oedema
E Muscle fasciculation

3.45 Under International Olympic Committee rules, which ONE of the following drugs would a competing athlete be able to take for the relief of a headache and cough?

A Terbutaline
B Phenylpropanolamine
C Co-proxamol
D Pseudoephedrine
E Mefenamic acid

3.46 A 24-year-old homosexual man with HIV infection is started on the drug zidovudine. Which ONE of the following statements about zidovudine therapy is TRUE?

A It is of proven benefit in HIV seroconversion syndromes
B It is metabolized principally in the kidney
C After conversion to zidovudine triphosphate, it inhibits HIV reverse transcriptase
D It slows the progression of clinical disease in asymptomatic HIV infection
E It reduces the infectivity of HIV infected individuals

3.47 **A 27-year-old woman is admitted for the treatment of a severe paracetamol overdose. Which ONE of the following statements about her management is TRUE?**
 A   Gastric lavage is useful up to 12 hours after the overdose
 B   Intravenous acetylcysteine is ineffective after 8 hours have elapsed since overdose
 C   Liver transplantation for acute hepatic failure is contraindicated
 D   Oral methionine is reserved for those presenting after 16 hours
 E   Wheeze is a recognized side-effect of N-acetylcysteine infusion

3.48 **Which ONE of the following statements about anti-arrhythmic drug therapy is TRUE?**
 A   Mexiletine is a class Ib anti-arrhythmic agent and delays the depolarization phase
 B   Adenosine is indicated in ventricular tachycardia
 C   Amiodarone is a class III anti-arrhythmic agent which shortens the duration of the action potential
 D   Verapamil is a class II anti-arrhythmic agent and inhibits the fast sodium channel
 E   Phenytoin accelerates conduction in Purkinje fibres

3.49 **Which ONE of the following statements about misoprostol therapy is TRUE?**
 A   It can be safely used in pregnant women
 B   It decreases the rate of peptic ulcer healing associated with NSAID therapy
 C   It produces abdominal pain and diarrhoea
 D   It promotes gastric acid secretion
 E   It is more effective than proton pump inhibitor therapy in preventing NSAID-induced gastropathy

3.50 **A 40-year-old woman has a renal transplant and is commenced on ciclosporin therapy. Which ONE of the following is LEAST likely to be due to ciclosporin toxicity?**
 A   Hypomagnesaemia
 B   Hypertrichosis
 C   Pulmonary infiltrates
 D   Gum hypertrophy
 E   Convulsions

ANSWERS

3.1　A　✗
　　　B　✗
　　　C　✗
　　　D　✔　May cause myopathy in toxic doses
　　　E　✗

3.2　A　✔　Acts on NMDA receptors
　　　B　✗
　　　C　✗　Competitive but irreversible
　　　D　✗　But does have partial agonist activity
　　　E　✗　Competes

3.3　A　✗　Rare but make provoke seizures in susceptible individuals
　　　B　✗　Well recognized, and especially in overdose or if given i.v.
　　　C　✗　May provoke seizures too
　　　D　✔
　　　E　✗　Lowers the seizure threshold

3.4　A　✗
　　　B　✗　This is just a measure of the shift in the dose response curve
　　　C　✗　A characteristic feature. It means that the maximum agonist response can still be achieved if enough agonist is added
　　　D　✗　Covalent binding is a feature of irreversible antagonists
　　　E　✔　It does not alter this property

3.5　A　✗　Usually sigmoidal if doses are plotted on a log scale
　　　B　✗　Calculated from a plot of fractional occupancy against dose
　　　C　✗　Irreversible antagonists are unsurmountable, so reduce the maximum response that can be obtained
　　　D　✔
　　　E　✗　This is a measure of efficacy, left-right variations in the dose response curve relate to potency

3.6　A　✗　Also ethanol and ethylene glycol
　　　B　✗
　　　C　✔　Desferrioxamine may be used
　　　D　✗
　　　E　✗

3.7　A　✗
　　　B　✗
　　　C　✔　Levels can be measured but their relationship with therapeutic response is poor
　　　D　✗
　　　E　✗

3.8   A   ✔   But may cause cough and angio-oedema
      B   ✘
      C   ✘
      D   ✘   Also busulfan, melphalan and cyclophosphamide
      E   ✘

3.9   A   ✔   Any drug whose pathway involves a major oxidative pathway is likely to induce haemolysis in individuals with G6PD deficiency. Other classical precipitants include dapsone, promaquine, sulphapyridine, acidosis and infection
      B   ✘
      C   ✘
      D   ✘
      E   ✘

3.10   A   ✘   Inhibit HMG CoA reductase and decrease LDL catabolism
      B   ✘   Decrease plasma LDL and cholesterol
      C   ✘   Decreases lipolysis and plasma triglycerides but increases plasma HDL
      D   ✘   Decrease plasma triglycerides and plasma LDL and increase plasma HDL
      E   ✔   Like colestyramine, it blocks bile acid reabsorption in the gut

3.11   A   ✘
      B   ✘
      C   ✘
      D   ✔   Stimulates satiety and can help some patients lose weight
      E   ✘   Increases insulin secretion

3.12   A   ✘   Well-known enzyme inducer, which increases the metabolism of oestrogens in the combined OCP, thus reducing its efficacy
      B   ✘   Enzyme induction
      C   ✔
      D   ✘   Altered bowel flora accelerates the enterohepatic elimination of sex hormones
      E   ✘   Enzyme induction

3.13   A   ✘   Usually presents with ataxia, coma, rarely fits and bradycardia
      B   ✘   May cause seizures, impaired consciousness, and dysrhythmias but not prolonged PR interval
      C   ✔   All typical TCA features
      D   ✘   Dysrhythmias are unusual
      E   ✘

3.14 A ✘ Approximately 1:10
     B ✘ It increases due to inhibition of negative feedback from angiotensin II
     C ✘ If anything, potassium levels may increase slightly
     D ✔ This is probably an important additional property of ACEi
     E ✘ This is a problem mainly in patients with heart failure in whom the renin angiotensin system is particularly activated

3.15 A ✘ Impaired renal function
     B ✔ Teratogenic in the first trimester and dangerous in late pregnancy due to increased risk of foetal bleeding during birth
     C ✘ May induce abortion
     D ✘ Damages teeth and bones
     E ✘ Marrow toxicity

3.16 A ✘ Increases by about 20%
     B ✘ Decreased due to the fall in plasma albumin concentration
     C ✘ Increased due to the increase in GFR
     D ✘ Unaltered unless vomiting is persistent
     E ✔ Typically increases due to enzyme induction rather than increased blood flow

3.17 A ✘ 'Desbrisoquine type' hydroxylation. Other drugs include codeine, flecainide, metoprolol, nortriptyline, perhexiline, and propafenone
     B ✘ Aceytylation by N-acetyltransferase (NAT2). Bimodal distribution in the population. Other drugs affected include hydralazine, procainamide and dapsone
     C ✔ Atenolol metabolism is not genetically determined
     D ✘ Catabolized by pseudoacetylcholinesterase (reduced activity in some individuals)
     E ✘ A hydroxylation reaction

3.18 A ✘
     B ✔ Dilated pupils are usual
     C ✘
     D ✘ Produces a syndrome similar to neuroleptic malignant syndrome
     E ✘ Metabolic acidosis may occur

3.19 A ✔ But cimetidine reduces the clearance of animophylline
     B ✘ Increases clearance, therefore higher dose may be required
     C ✘ Reduced clearance
     D ✘ Reduced clearance
     E ✘ Omit loading dose

3.20 A ✔
     B ✘ Phase I usually involves healthy volunteers and phase II patients
     C ✘ All adverse events should be recorded and included in the final report
     D ✘ Red is the most efficacious colour and yellow the least
     E ✘ 'First-in-man' studies are typically non-randomized, escalating dose studies

3.21 A ✘ Inhibitory effect
     B ✘ Vigabatrin inhibits GABA aminotransferase and enzymes that degrade GABA, an inhibitory neurotransmitter
     C ✔
     D ✘ Inhibitory effect hence value of combining L-dopa with co-carbidopa in the treatment of Parkinson's disease
     E ✘ Inhibitory effect

3.22 A ✘ Flumazenil; use with caution as it may provoke seizures in tricyclic poisoning
     B ✘ Fomepizole or ethanol
     C ✘ Dicobalt edetate; methylene blue is used in the treatment of methaemoglobinaemia
     D ✔ Useful to treat and/or prevent seizures
     E ✘ Atropine; thioctic acid is used in *Amanita* poisoning

3.23 A ✘ All serious reactions should be reported to the Committee of Safety of Medicines (CSM) in the UK. However, well-recognized minor reactions need not be reported except for new drugs or those of particular interest — indicated by a black triangle in the BNF.
     B ✘
     C ✘
     D ✔ But it is good clinical practice
     E ✘ Far fewer than half

3.24 A ✘ Reduces lithium excretion and may provoke toxicity
     B ✘ Can cause methotrexate toxicity by blocking its excretion
     C ✔ Sometimes used to increase plasma penicillin levels to enhance therapeutic effect
     D ✘ Ciprofloxacin inhibits the metabolism of warfarin, potentiating its anticoagulant effect, but does not alter renal excretion
     E ✘ Reduces renal clearance of digoxin

3.25 A ✘ Common
     B ✘
     C ✘ Hyperthyroidism is more common though
     D ✘ Thought to be due to demyelination
     E ✔

3.26 A ✗ This means that the rate of metabolism does not change as more drug is given. Thus small increases in dose can have dramatic effects on plasma concentration and thus adverse events

B ✗

C ✗

D ✔ But verapamil does have zero-order kinetics

E ✗

3.27 A ✗

B ✔ Avoid due to risk of metabolic acidosis

C ✗

D ✗

E ✗

3.28 A ✗ In about 5–10% of asthmatics — 'aspirin-sensitive asthma'

B ✔

C ✗ Usually a direct irritant effect

D ✗ Aspirin-sensitive asthmatics are also sensitive to NSAIDs and some food colourings and salicylates in foodstuffs

E ✗ Parasympathomimetics may aggravate asthma

3.29 A ✗ Hypertensive crisis and tachycardia

B ✗ Adrenocortical insufficiency and increased disease activity

C ✗ Supersensitivity of beta-adrenergic receptors may result in hypertensive crisis and severe angina or myocardial infarction

D ✗ Confusion, convulsions and conditions resembling delirium tremens

E ✔ No adverse effects following withdrawal

3.30 A ✗ The bioavailability of any drug is expressed as the ratio of the area under the absorption curve after oral/parenteral administration. Any factor that delays drug absorption or entry into the systemic circulation will therefore adversely affect its bioavailability

B ✗

C ✗

D ✔

E ✗

3.31 A ✗ Inherited as an autosomal dominant trait, the condition may be linked with other myotonic disorders. Intracellular transport of calcium is deranged and generalized muscular contraction may be provoked by many agents

B ✗

C ✗

D ✗

E ✔ May be used in the treatment of the condition

3.32 A ✘
     B ✘ Metal ions do not bind to charcoal
     C ✔
     D ✘ Convulsions occur and are treated with diazepam
     E ✘

3.33 A ✘ Inhibits leucocyte migration and the production of
         leucotactic factors
     B ✘ It has no effect on urate clearance
     C ✘ But useful in the treatment of familial Mediterranean fever
     D ✔ Usually effective within 6 hours of administration
     E ✘ Nausea, vomiting, abdominal pain and diarrhoea are
         common

3.34 A ✔ Drugs stimulating microsomal enzyme induction will
         precipitate symptoms
     B ✘ Drugs known to be safe include penicillin, pethidine,
         diazepam, diamorphine, acetylsalicylic acid and
         chlorpromazine
     C ✘ Erythropoietic porphyrias are not aggravated by drug
         therapy other than drugs which induce photosensitivity
     D ✘
     E ✘

3.35 A ✘ Usually the immune complex of the drug and
         immunoglobulin attaches to the red blood cells. In
         contrast, penicillin binds directly to the RBCs
     B ✘
     C ✘
     D ✘
     E ✔

3.36 A ✔ Isoniazid toxicity is usually related to dose and acetylator
         status
     B ✘
     C ✘ Because of bacterial resistance, triple therapy is always
         necessary
     D ✘ Pyrazinamide and isoniazid penetrate the CSF
     E ✘ It produces hepatocellular jaundice

3.37 A ✘ Usually associated with very high blood lead levels
     B ✘ Metallic taste in the mouth and colic are the earliest
         features
     C ✔ Microcytic, hypochromic anaemia with basophilic stippling
     D ✘ Saturnine gout due to renal insufficiency
     E ✘ Motor neuropathy is more common than sensory
         neuropathy

3.38 A ✔ 50% have recently consumed alcohol; clinical features can be difficult
     B ✗ At least 50% of such patients have a history of multiple drug overdosages
     C ✗ Only a minority express suicidal intent
     D ✗
     E ✗

3.39 A ✔ Strong acid and alkali solutions will produce corrosive mouth changes
     B ✗ Circulatory collapse and metabolic acidosis may occur within 12–24 hours
     C ✗ Haemorrhagic gastroenteritis is common, resulting in vomiting, diarrhoea, abdominal pain and gastrointestinal bleeding
     D ✗ Lassitude and drowsiness indicate serious poisoning with encephalopathy
     E ✗

3.40 A ✗ Acute gout may respond dramatically to corticosteroid therapy
     B ✗ Increases BP but steroid therapy is unlikely to be prolonged
     C ✗ Disseminated varicella is unlikely unless the patient has shingles
     D ✔ Corneal ulceration may progress rapidly
     E ✗ The effect is modest and can be avoided with PPI therapy

3.41 A ✗ Due to the impaired peripheral glucose uptake, hyperinsulinism and inhibition of gluconeogenesis (diabetics are at special risk)
     B ✗ By the inhibition of hepatic lactate uptake and gluconeogenesis
     C ✗ Inhibits the secretion of antidiuretic hormone promoting a diuresis; the resulting thirst may produce water intoxication post-diuresis
     D ✔ Chronic alcohol abuse may produce a congestive cardiomyopathy
     E ✗ False-localizing neurological signs including respiratory depression

3.42 A ✗ Well absorbed and oxidized to formaldehyde and formic acid
     B ✗ Toxicity results from formic acid formation
     C ✔ Ethyl alcohol retards the oxidation of methanol
     D ✗ Metabolic acidosis requiring intravenous fluid and alkali therapy
     E ✗ Treatment with ethyl alcohol and/or haemodialysis should prevent blindness which is due to the effect of formaldehyde on the retinal cells

3.43   A   ✗   Interferes with purine biosynthesis
      B   ✔   Dihydrofolate reductase inhibitor, so affects purines <u>and</u> pyrimidines
      C   ✗   Interferes with microtubule assembly, causing metaphase arrest
      D   ✗   Inhibits DNA topoisomerase II action
      E   ✗   An alkylating agent

3.44   A   ✔   Cholinesterase inhibition produces small pupils
      B   ✗
      C   ✗   All cholinergic effects
      D   ✗
      E   ✗

3.45   A   ✗
      B   ✗   Nasal decongestants often contain banned sympathomimetic agents
      C   ✗   Contains dextropropoxyphene — an opioid
      D   ✗
      E   ✔

3.46   A   ✗   May give symptomatic relief in some patients with neuropathy
      B   ✗   60–80% by glucuronidation in the liver
      C   ✔   Prevents viral replication in newly infected cells
      D   ✗   No long-term benefit
      E   ✗

3.47   A   ✗   Gastric lavage useful up to 4 hours after ingestion
      B   ✗   Can be used for up to 24 hours in encephalopathic patients
      C   ✗   Specialist advice should be sought
      D   ✗
      E   ✔   A pseudo-anaphylactoid reaction

3.48   A   ✔   Orally effective and not as rapidly metabolized as lidocaine (lignocaine)
      B   ✗   Useful in SVTs including those associated with accessory pathways
      C   ✗   Prolongs the duration of the action potential; it has a long half-life (30 days); useful in WPW syndrome. Side-effects include thyroid dysfunction, photosensitization and corneal deposits
      D   ✗   Class IV agent inhibiting the slow calcium channel. Class I agents like lidocaine (lignocaine) inhibit the fast sodium channel
      E   ✗   Useful in ventricular arrhythmias associated with digoxin or hypokalaemia

3.49 A ✗ Increases uterine contractility and causes miscarriage
B ✗ Accelerates healing and helps prevent NSAID gastropathy
C ✔ The commonest side-effect
D ✗ Inhibits gastric acid secretion and improves cytoprotection
E ✗ Less effective than PPIs in protecting the stomach and
duodenum

3.50 A ✗
B ✗
C ✔ Commonly reported with azathioprine therapy
D ✗
E ✗

4

Gastroenterology and hepatology

QUESTIONS

4.1 **Which ONE of the following statements about the neuroendocrine control of the alimentary tract is TRUE?**
A Mucosal secretion is mediated by neuropeptides
B The initial release of gastrin occurs in response to gastric distension
C Sympathetic nerve fibres run in the pelvic nerves
D Parasympathetic stimuli mediate the inhibition of secretin secretion
E Somatostatin induces the secretion of upper GI hormones

4.2 **Which ONE of the following statements about the normal alimentary tract is TRUE?**
A Mucosa-associated lymphoid tissue constitutes 75% of the total body lymphatic tissue
B Secretory IgM protects the gut from bacterial invasion
C Water-soluble drugs enter the portal and systemic circulations via lymphatics
D Folic acid is chiefly absorbed in the terminal ileum
E Exocrine pancreatic secretion is controlled principally by hormonal factors

4.3 **Which ONE of the following statements about the normal digestive processes is TRUE?**
A Small bowel contractile activity ceases during fasting
B Triglycerides are hydrolysed to monoglycerides by the effects of secretin
C Disaccharides are absorbed by an active process and metabolized in the liver
D Pancreatic trypsinogen is stimulated by the release of cholecystokinin
E Colonic motility is principally controlled by the hormone motilin

4.4 **A 45-year-old man presents with bilateral enlargement of the salivary glands. Which ONE of the following disorders is LEAST LIKELY to be responsible?**
A Alcoholic liver disease
B Sjögren's syndrome
C Bacterial infection
D Sarcoidosis
E Measles virus infection

4.5 **A 56-year-old woman presents with dysphagia and an iron deficiency anaemia associated with a pharyngeal pouch. Which ONE of the following statements is TRUE?**
   A Fibreoptic gastroscopy is the investigation of choice rather than a barium meal
   B Dysphagia is likely to be localized to the mid-sternum
   C The presentation is unusual as most patients present in early adolescence
   D There is a significant risk of recurrent pneumonia
   E Dysphagia is typically rapidly progressive

4.6 **A 60-year-old man presents to the casualty department with central chest pain. The ECG and serum troponin are normal and a diagnosis of diffuse oesophageal spasm is suspected. Which ONE of the following statements is TRUE?**
   A Oesophageal histology is likely to reveal an abnormal Auerbach's plexus
   B Most patients are likely to present before the age of 40 years
   C Oesophageal motility studies are likely to reveal spontaneous coordinated contractions
   D Dysphagia is usually attributable to an associated oesophagitis
   E Acid-lowering drug therapy is unlikely to reduce the frequency of chest pain

4.7 **Which ONE of the following is a typical feature of a gastrinoma?**
   A A small gastric tumour
   B Absence of hepatic metastases at presentation
   C Thyroid adenomas
   D Constipation rather than diarrhoea
   E Absent acid secretory response to pentagastrin stimulation

4.8 **Which ONE of the following satatements about the blind loop syndrome is TRUE?**
   A The finding of 10^3 coliform organisms/ml in the duodenal aspirate is diagnostic
   B A macrocytic anaemia is typically due to folate deficiency
   C The finding of steatorrhoea suggests the problem is pancreatic in origin
   D The diagnosis is best confirmed using the SeHCAT absorption test
   E The absence of serum IgA raises the possibility of giardiasis

4.9 **A 50-year-old man with weight loss and chronic diarrhoea is suspected of having a malabsorption syndrome. In which ONE of the following disorders would the finding of subtotal villous atrophy on small bowel biopsy suggest an unrelated diagnosis?**
   A Dermatitis herpetiformis
   B Whipple's disease
   C Zollinger–Ellison syndrome
   D Immerslund–Grasbeck syndrome
   E Tropical sprue

4.10 In a patient with Whipple's disease, which ONE of the following clinical features suggests an alternative or additional disease?
A Chronic renal failure
B Peripheral arthritis
C Pericarditis and myocarditis
D Cranial nerve palsies
E Meningitis

4.11 In which ONE of the following diagnoses would the finding of a protein-losing enteropathy suggest an alternative diagnosis?
A Abetalipoproteinaemia
B Radiation enteritis
C Intestinal lymphoma
D Ménétrier's disease
E Intestinal lymphangiectasia

4.12 Which ONE of the following statements about pancreas divisum is TRUE?
A It occurs with a prevalence rate of about 1% in the normal population
B It results in both acute but not chronic pancreatitis
C It represents a failure of fusion of the embryonic dorsal and ventral ducts
D Gastric outlet obstruction is a recognized complication of the anomaly
E An association with malrotation of the foregut is a common finding

4.13 A 24-year-old man presents with severe diarrhoea, urgency of defecation and rectal bleeding; a diagnosis of acute ulcerative colitis is suspected. Which ONE of the following statements about the management of this man is TRUE?
A Antibiotic therapy is mandatory if the patient is febrile
B Antidiarrhoeal agents increase the risk of toxic dilatation
C Systemic corticosteroids should induce a remission in all patients
D Hypoproteinaemia is an indication for parenteral albumin infusion
E Progressive colonic dilatation despite medical therapy requires infliximab therapy

4.14 In the maintenance treatment of ulcerative colitis, which ONE of the following statements is TRUE?
A Corticosteroid therapy should be given orally rather than rectally
B Aminosalicylate therapy reduces the risk of colonic carcinoma
C Azathioprine therapy is contraindicated if maintenance corticosteroid is required
D The development of renal impairment suggests aminosalicylate toxicity
E Aminosalicylate therapy is effective only if given by mouth

4.15 **Which ONE of the following complications is more likely to occur in association with ulcerative colitis than with Crohn's disease?**
A   Vitamin B_{12} deficiency
B   Erythema nodosum
C   Enteropathic arthritis
D   Aphthous mouth ulcers
E   Small bowel lymphoma

4.16 **A 22-year-old woman with recurrent abdominal pain is found to have ileocaecal Crohn's disease on the barium follow through examination. Which ONE of the following is TRUE?**
A   Surgical bypass is preferable to a limited bowel resection
B   Stopping smoking reduces the risk of symptomatic relapses
C   Corticosteroid therapy is contraindicated in the acute phase
D   Colestyramine reduces the diarrhoea by decreasing the steatorrhoea
E   Aminosalicylate therapy reduces the risk of small bowel obstruction

4.17 **Which ONE of the statements about subacute colonic obstruction is TRUE?**
A   Vomiting is often an early feature
B   The finding of an empty rectum usually excludes faecal impaction
C   Quiet bowel sounds exclude mechanical obstruction
D   Persisting diarrhoea excludes obstruction
E   Abdominal tenderness suggests strangulation or peritonitis

4.18 **Which ONE of the following statements about Hirschsprung's disease of the colon is TRUE?**
A   There is a family history in 90% of cases
B   Presentation typically occurs between the ages of 3 and 5 years
C   There is a segmental absence of the myenteric nerve plexus
D   The rectum is typically loaded on digital examination
E   The surgical treatment of choice is a defunctioning colostomy

4.19 **Which ONE of the following statements about colonic polyps is TRUE?**
A   75% of polyps occur in the right hemicolon
B   The typical histology is that of tubular adenoma
C   Polyps <2 cm in diameter are usually malignant
D   Intussusception is a recognized complication
E   Presentation with colonic bleeding is typical

4.20 **Which ONE of the following statements about colonic carcinoma is TRUE?**
A It is the commonest of all carcinomas in the UK
B The majority of carcinomas arise in the right hemicolon
C After resection, there is a recognized risk of a second carcinoma
D Dukes' A classifies tumour extending to the serosa only
E Only a minority of rectal tumours are palpable per rectum

4.21 **Which ONE of the following facts about the normal liver is TRUE?**
A The space of Disse separates the biliary ductules from the portal venules
B The hepatic artery supplies 50% of the total hepatic oxygen supply
C Kupffer cells are derived from blood neutrophil leucocytes
D Stellate (Ito) cells are responsible for the uptake and storage of vitamin K
E The liver is subdivided into 11 segments based on the hepatic blood supply

4.22 **Which ONE of the following statements about liver function tests is TRUE?**
A The albumin concentration falls rapidly within the first 3 days of acute liver failure
B Persistent hypergammaglobulinaemia indicates hepatocyte necrosis
C An increased IgG concentration is typical of alcoholic hepatitis
D The prothrombin time increases rapidly in severe acute hepatitis
E An increased IgG concentration suggests primary biliary cirrhosis

4.23 **A 16-year-old female presents with jaundice and dark urine. The serum alkaline phosphatase, and γ glutamyl transpeptidase are markedly raised but the serum alanine aminotransferase is only marginally raised. Ultrasound examination reveals extrahepatic biliary obstruction. Which ONE of the following is the most likely diagnosis?**
A Sclerosing cholangitis
B Primary biliary cirrhosis
C Cystic fibrosis
D Alcoholic cirrhosis
E Non-alcoholic steatohepatitis

4.24 A 21-year-old male presents with acute nausea, vomiting and abdominal pain. The liver function tests reveal marginal elevation of the serum alkaline phosphatase but the serum alanine aminotransferase is raised at ten times the normal value. Ultrasound examination reveals no evidence of biliary tract obstruction and a screen for viral and autoimmune hepatitis is negative. Given the persistence of nausea and markedly deranged serum liver function values 3 months later, a liver biopsy is undertaken. Which ONE of the following pathological changes best characterizes the diagnosis of acute hepatitis?

A Polymorph leucocyte infiltration of the lobules
B Sparing of the centrilobular areas
C Obliteration of the portal tracts
D Hepatocyte necrosis with deeply-stained acidophilic bodies
E Fatty infiltration

4.25 A 45-year-old woman presents with a 1 year history of itching and the recent onset of jaundice associated with marked elevation of the serum alkaline phosphatase. A liver biopsy is undertaken. Which ONE of the following pathological changes best characterizes the diagnosis of primary biliary cirrhosis?

A Lymphocyte invasion of the portal–periportal interface
B Periportal hepatocytic damage with the formation of 'rosettes'
C Absence of hepatic granulomata
D Proliferation of the portal venules
E Lymphocyte infiltration of the portal triads

4.26 Which ONE of the following statements about hepatitis D (HDV) is TRUE?

A The infective agent is a DNA virus
B Transmission is usually via the enteral route
C Replication of the virus requires the presence of the hepatitis A virus
D Delta virus particles often persist in the blood for many years
E Pre-existing hepatitis B carriage predisposes to the progression to cirrhosis

4.27 Which ONE of the following statements about hepatitis E (HEV) is TRUE?

A The infective agent is a DNA virus
B The principal mode of transmission is via the parenteral route
C The incubation period is 3–6 months
D If infection is acquired during pregnancy, acute hepatitis is more likely to develop
E Chronic hepatitis similar to that seen in hepatitis B infection is a likely outcome

4.28 A 35-year-old woman presents with an acute confusional state and vomiting, having been well 5 days previously. On examination, she is jaundiced associated with subconjunctival haemorrhages, foetor and dark brown urine. Liver function tests reveal a plasma bilirubin 180 μmol/L, ALT 9,500 iu/L and the prothrombin ratio 3.4. Which ONE of the following investigations is of the LEAST diagnostic value?
   A   Serum ferritin concentration
   B   Serum caeruloplasmin concentration
   C   Anti-hepatitis A and B antibody titres
   D   Urinary and plasma paracetamol concentrations
   E   Ultrasound scan of the liver

4.29 Which ONE of the following features of chronic hepatitis due to hepatitis B infection differs MOST from the features of autoimmune hepatitis?
   A   Typically affects females
   B   Often produces acute hepatic failure
   C   Is characterized by florid physical signs
   D   Typically progresses slowly without exacerbations
   E   Is less likely to be complicated by hepatoma

4.30 Eight weeks after the onset of an acute hepatitis, which ONE the following serum tests strongly suggests an alternative diagnosis to that of autoimmune hepatitis?
   A   Antinuclear and smooth muscle antibodies in high titres
   B   High titres of anti-LKM antibodies
   C   Hypoalbuminaemia with hypergammaglobulinaemia
   D   Increased ferritin concentration
   E   Anti-mitochondrial antibody titre >640

4.31 Which ONE of the following statements about the management of a patient with autoimmune hepatitis is TRUE?
   A   Liver biopsy should be undertaken as soon as possible after the onset of the illness
   B   Remissions and relapses are characteristic
   C   Associated with autoantibodies, 50% of patients die within 5 years despite treatment
   D   Corticosteroid and azathioprine therapy should not be used in combination
   E   Interferon is of proven value in neonatally-acquired chronic type B viral hepatitis

4.32 Which ONE of the following statements about hepatic cirrhosis in the UK is TRUE?

A No cause is found in 60% of patients

B It develops as an early complication of severe acute type B viral hepatitis

C It is a recognized complication of acute paracetamol poisoning

D 90% of patients with chronic alcohol abuse eventually develop cirrhosis

E It is a recognized complication of protein calorie malnutrition

4.33 A 68-year-old homeless man is admitted with lethargy and mild jaundice. He admits to drinking a litre of vodka a day for several years. An ultrasound scan shows marked nodularity of the liver and ascites. Which ONE of the following statements is TRUE?

A Central cyanosis, if present, should respond to 40% oxygen therapy

B An increasing serum alkaline phosphatase suggests progressive liver failure

C Peripheral blood flow is likely to be reduced

D Glomerular filtration rate is likely to be increased

E The presence of ascites is likely to be the result of portal hypertension

4.34 In which ONE of the following disorders would the development of hepatic cirrhosis suggest an additional or alternative diagnosis to explain the liver disease?

A Haemochromatosis

B Wilson's disease

C Macrovesicular hepatosteatosis

D Hepatitis C infection

E Alpha$_1$-antitrypsin deficiency

4.35 A 55-year-old man with chronic liver failure due to alcoholic liver disease presents with an acute confusional state. On examination, he has a flapping tremor, foetor and ascites. Which ONE of his current drug therapies is LEAST likely to be contributing to acute hepatic decompensation?

A Spironolactone

B Furosemide (frusemide)

C Naproxen

D Loperamide

E Amoxicillin

4.36 **Which ONE of the following statements about the management of severe acute hepatic encephalopathy is TRUE?**
A   Dietary protein intake should be restricted to 60 g per day
B   The use of sedatives is recommended to minimize neuropsychiatric symptoms
C   Neomycin therapy should be given to reduce colonic bacterial fermentation
D   Diuretic therapy often helps to prevent the development of cerebral oedema
E   Enteral or parenteral glucose up to 300 g/day should be administered

4.37 **Which ONE of the following features best characterizes the hepatorenal syndrome in cirrhosis?**
A   Acute renal tubular necrosis
B   Proteinuria and an abnormal urinary sediment
C   Urinary sodium concentration <10 mmol/L
D   Urine/plasma osmolality ratio <1.0
E   An elevated central venous pressure in most patients

4.38 **Which ONE of the following statements about the management of ascites due to hepatic cirrhosis is TRUE?**
A   The dietary sodium intake should be restricted to 80 mmol/day
B   Paracentesis and parenteral albumin replacement improves the survival rate
C   The daily calorie intake should be restricted to 1500 calories
D   Diuretic therapy should achieve a daily weight loss of at least 2.5 kg
E   The protein intake should be at least 60 g/day unless encephalopathy is suspected

4.39 **Which ONE of the following features is most compatible with a diagnosis of primary biliary cirrhosis?**
A   Xanthomata affecting the palmar creases and eyelids
B   Death from liver failure within 5 years of the diagnosis
C   Splenomegaly preceding the development of hepatomegaly
D   Dilated bile ducts on ultrasonography
E   Improved survival rate with immunosuppressant therapy

4.40 **Which ONE of the following findings indicates the need to consider orthotopic liver transplantation in a patient with chronic liver failure due to alcoholic cirrhosis?**
A   Serum bilirubin 45 mmol/L
B   Hyponatraemia complicating diuretic therapy
C   Encephalopathy resistant to medical therapy
D   Arterial hypoxaemia associated with chronic respiratory failure
E   Presence of a 10 cm hepatoma in a cirrhotic liver

4.41 **Which ONE of the following statements about the biliary tract is TRUE?**
A The right and left hepatic ducts join to form the common bile duct
B The normal common bile duct measures 25 mm in diameter
C The bile and pancreatic ducts usually join the duodenum separately
D The gallbladder is mainly innervated by sympathetic nerves
E 1–2 litres of bile are secreted daily and concentrated 10-fold in the gallbladder

4.42 **Which ONE of the following statements about gallstones is TRUE?**
A More common in Africa and in India than in Europe
B Demonstrable in over 80% of UK patients >60 years of age
C Predominantly composed of bile pigment in most gallstones in the UK
D Usually pigment stones in hepatic cirrhosis
E Usually the result of reduced hepatic bile acid secretion

4.43 **Which ONE of the following features is MOST typical of acute cholecystitis?**
A The absence of obstruction of the cystic duct
B Sterile culture of bile 72 hours after onset
C An invariable association with gallstones
D Exacerbation of pain following morphine analgesics
E Absence of apparent gallstones on plain X-ray

4.44 **Which ONE of the following features would be an expected finding in cholangiocarcinoma?**
A Association with hepatic cirrhosis
B Abdominal pain and obstructive jaundice
C High titres of serum alpha-fetoprotein
D Minor elevation of the serum alkaline phosphatase
E Surgically resectable in the majority of cases

4.45 **Which ONE of the following statements about carcinoma of the gallbladder is TRUE?**
A The disorder is much commoner in males than females
B The tumour is usually squamous cell in type
C The disorder is typically associated with longstanding gallstones
D The plasma CA-125 is characteristically markedly increased
E Curative surgical resection is usually possible in most instances

ANSWERS

4.1 A ✔ Vasoactive intestinal peptide and substance P
    B ✘ The thought or smell of food induces a vagally-mediated response
    C ✘ Run in the splanchnic nerves to the myenteric and submucous plexuses
    D ✘ Vagus stimulates secretion
    E ✘ Inhibits secretion of many of the GI hormones

4.2 A ✘ 25% of the total body lymphatic tissue and an important defence mechanism
    B ✘ Secretory IgA synthesized by B lymphocytes
    C ✘ Fat-soluble drugs and vitamins together with chylomicrons and lipoproteins
    D ✘ Actively absorbed throughout the entire small intestine
    E ✔ The autonomic nervous system is also involved

4.3 A ✘ Migrating motor complexes (MMC) traverse the small bowel every 1–2 hours
    B ✘ Lipase and colipase; secretin induces pancreatic secretion of bicarbonate
    C ✘ Digested by the mucosal disaccharidase enzymes lactase, sucrase and maltase
    D ✔ Trypsinogen is activated to trypsin by duodenal enterokinase
    E ✘ The autonomic nervous system, neuropeptides and other hormones

4.4 A ✘ Also associated with malnutrition and autoimmune hepatitis
    B ✘ Associated with dry mouth and kerotoconjunctivitis sicca (dry eyes)
    C ✘ May be associated with calculi in the parotid duct
    D ✘ Uveoparotid fever (Heerdfordt's syndrome)
    E ✔ Typically associated with mumps virus infection

4.5 A ✘ May be hazardous due to inadvertent perforation
    B ✘ Characteristically associated with regurgitation
    C ✘ Typically presents in later life
    D ✔ Due to recurrent aspiration
    E ✘ Dysphagia only progresses very slowly

4.6 A ✘ But there are degenerative changes in the vagal nerve
    B ✘ Usually over the age of 60 but presentation can be at any age
    C ✘ Uncoordinated contractions occur sometimes in response to emotional arousal
    D ✘ Uncoordinated contractions per se may cause dysphagia
    E ✔ Only if the contractions are associated with acid reflux

4.7 A ✗ Tumour is usually in the pancreas or duodenum
B ✗ 50% of tumours have metastasized at presentation
C ✗ Parathyroid adenomas occur in 30–60% (multiple endocrine neoplasia MEN type 1)
D ✗ 40% of patients with the Zollinger–Ellison syndrome have diarrhoea
E ✔ Acid secretion is already maximally stimulated

4.8 A ✗ Often > 10^8 coliform organisms/ml
B ✗ Usually due to vitamin B_{12} deficiency
C ✗ Due to deconjugation of bile acids
D ✗ ^{14}C-glycocholate breath test
E ✔ And gluten enteropathy

4.9 A ✗ Most patients have an associated gluten enteropathy
B ✗ Rare infection with Gram-positive bacilli *Tropheryma whippelli*
C ✗
D ✔ Congenital abnormality of the terminal ileal receptor for intrinsic factor
E ✗ Small bowel infection in the Caribbean and in Asia particularly

4.10 A ✔ Can affect almost every other organ
B ✗ Usually peripheral joints, occasionally the sacroiliac joints
C ✗ Also fever and lymphadenopathy
D ✗ Produces a characteristic disorder of ocular movements
E ✗ Gram-positive bacilli *Tropheryma whippelli*

4.11 A ✔ Produces fat malabsorption
B ✗
C ✗ And gluten enteropathy
D ✗
E ✗ And constrictive pericarditis

4.12 A ✗ Prevalence rate 7–10%
B ✗ Acute and chronic pancreatic drainage is via the smaller accessory ampulla
C ✔
D ✗ This can occur in annular pancreas
E ✗ This and gut atresias are associated with annular pancreas

4.13 A ✗ Pyrexia results from the inflammatory process
B ✔ Loperamide and codeine phosphate are best avoided in the acute situation
C ✗ Some patients require urgent surgery
D ✗ Indication for nutritional support but improves as the disease improves
E ✗ These patients need urgent surgery

4.14   A   ✗   Oral steroids are reserved for more active disease
      B   ✗   Reduces the rate of relapse
      C   ✗   'Steroid-sparing' effect helps minimize adverse effects
      D   ✔   Causes interstitial nephritis; monitoring renal function is advisable
         ✗   Effective given orally or rectally

4.15   A   ✗   Due to terminal ileal disease
      B   ✗
      C   ✔   Seronegative spondyloarthritis
      D   ✗   Can be severe and herald the onset of Crohn's disease
      E   ✗

4.16   A   ✗   Stricturoplasty helps to limit the length of gut resected
      B   ✔   And reduces the likelihood of further surgery
      C   ✗   Intravenous hydrocortisone in severe active disease
      D   ✗   Binds bile salts and impairs fat absorption
      E   ✗   Major role is in colonic disease

4.17   A   ✗   Late or even absent in colonic obstruction
      B   ✗
      C   ✗   But absent bowel sounds suggest paralytic ileus
      D   ✗   Fluid stools can occur—'spurious' diarrhoea
      E   ✔   Usually with constant severe pain

4.18   A   ✗   Family history in 30% of cases
      B   ✗   Symptoms usually date from birth
      C   ✔   In the pelvic colon and rectum
      D   ✗   Rectum is empty
      E   ✗   Excision of the abnormal segment with colorectal anastomosis

4.19   A   ✗   Most occur in the left hemicolon
      B   ✗   And tubulovillous and villous adenomata
      C   ✗   >50% are malignant if >2 cm in size
      D   ✗   Causing mechanical bowel obstruction
      E   ✔   Bleeding or mucus discharge are common

4.20   A   ✗   Breast and lung carcinoma are more common; commonest GI malignancy
      B   ✗   75% occur in the left hemicolon
      C   ✔   Particularly in the presence of colonic polyps
      D   ✗   Spread not beyond muscularis
      E   ✗   Majority are palpable hence the need to do a PR examination

4.21 A ✗ Separates the hepatocytes from the endothelium
B ✔ But only 25% of hepatic blood flow
C ✗ Derived from monocytes and account for 80% of the body's phagocytic capacity
D ✗ Ito cells store vitamin A and also produce cytokines and collagenases
E ✗ Eight segments associated with the subdivisions of the hepatic and portal veins

4.22 A ✗ The half-life of serum albumin is about 20–26 days
B ✗ May reflect bypass of hepatic immune mechanisms
C ✗ An increased IgA concentration is more characteristic
D ✔ Half-lives of clotting factors 2, 7, 9 and 10 are short (5–72 hours)
E ✗ Typically an increased IgM level

4.23 A ✗ Intrahepatic
B ✗ Intrahepatic
C ✔ CBD obstruction from chronic pancreatitis
D ✗ Intrahepatic
E ✗ Rarely causes jaundice

4.24 A ✗ Mononuclear cell infiltrate 'lobulitis'
B ✗ These areas tend to be more affected
C ✗ Mononuclear cell infiltrate 'triaditis'
D ✔ Councilman bodies
E ✗ Seen in alcohol abuse and with other hepatotoxins

4.25 A ✗ Suggests interface hepatitis
B ✗ Classical feature of interface hepatitis
C ✗ Granulomatous change is common
D ✗ Proliferation of the biliary ductules
E ✔ And a biliary pattern of fibrosis

4.26 A ✗ An RNA-defective virus
B ✗ Transmitted like hepatitis B parenterally
C ✗ Incapable of replication without hepatitis B virus; incubation is 6–9 weeks
D ✗ Often only transiently detected and the anti-HDV titre is a more useful marker
E ✔ Hepatitis B may then resolve

4.27 A ✗ Infective agent is an RNA virus
B ✗ Principal mode of transmission is via the faecal–oral route
C ✗ Clinical illness resembles HAV infection with an incubation period of 3–8 weeks
D ✔
E ✗ Chronic hepatitis does not develop

4.28 A ✔ Elevated in most patients with fulminant hepatic failure
  B ✗ And serum and urinary copper to exclude Wilson's disease
  C ✗ Check IgM antibodies to hepatitis A, B, D; viral titres of EBV, CMV and HSV
  D ✗ Consider other drugs and poisons; check for autoimmune liver disease
  E ✗ And doppler USS of hepatic veins (Budd–Chiari syndrome)

4.29 A ✗ In contrast to autoimmune hepatitis
  B ✗ A chronically progressive course is more typical
  C ✗ Signs are sparse; hepatomegaly is common
  D ✔ Particularly if HBeAg present
  E ✗ Hepatoma is more common

4.30 A ✗ Found in 50–66% of patients with autoimmune hepatitis (AIH)
  B ✗ Type II AIH with microsomal antibodies to liver and kidney
  C ✗ In presence of elevated serum ALT levels
  D ✗ Often elevated in hepatitis irrespective of the aetiology
  E ✔ Suggests primary biliary cirrhosis

4.31 A ✗ Defer biopsy if possible for 6 months
  B ✔ Most ultimately develop cirrhosis
  C ✗ About 10% of patients die within 5 years despite treatment
  D ✗ Azathioprine also facilitates a reduction in corticosteroid therapy
  E ✗ Also of limited value in chronic type B viral hepatitis

4.32 A ✗ The majority of cases in the UK are alcohol related
  B ✔ Or a later complication of chronic infection
  C ✗ May cause acute massive hepatic necrosis
  D ✗ Develops in no more than 50% of patients
  E ✗ Produces a fatty liver (macrovesicular steatosis)

4.33 A ✗ In cirrhosis, refractory hypoxaemia results from intrapulmonary shunting
  B ✗ Increasing bilirubin, falling serum albumin and rising prothrombin time
  C ✗ Peripheral vasodilatation occurs
  D ✗ Visceral blood flow is generally reduced
  E ✔ As may oesophageal varices and splenomegaly

4.34 A ✗ Hepatoma is also likely to occur
  B ✗
  C ✔ Common and benign
  D ✗ HBV, HCV, HDV infections
  E ✗

4.35 A ✗ Hypovolaemia exacerbates encephalopathy
  B ✗ Hypokalaemia and hypovolaemia exacerbates encephalopathy
  C ✗ Prostaglandin synthesis inhibition reduces intrahepatic circulation
  D ✗ Constipation promotes colonic bacterial protein breakdown
  E ✔ May reduce colonic bacterial protein breakdown

4.36 A ✗ Should be reduced to less than 20 g per day
  B ✗ May worsen or precipitate encephalopathy
  C ✗ No better than placebo; may have a role in chronic encephalopathy
  D ✗ May be required for coexistent ascites but may worsen encephalopathy
  E ✔ Hypoglycaemia is a likely complication

4.37 A ✗ No intrinsic renal damage
  B ✗ Suggests glomerular disease
  C ✔ Normal renal response to secondary hyperaldosteronism
  D ✗ Ratio >1.5
  E ✗ Hypovolaemia is more common

4.38 A ✗ Restriction <40 mmol/day is usually required
  B ✗ A palliative, symptomatic measure with no prognostic value
  C ✗ Calorie restriction is neither required nor desirable
  D ✗ Weight loss >1 kg/day may precipitate renal impairment and/or encephalopathy
  E ✔ Restriction may be necessary to control encephalopathy

4.39 A ✔ And on elbows, knees and buttocks
  B ✗ Prognosis excellent in the absence of symptoms or signs
  C ✗ Splenomegaly occurs after the development of portal hypertension
  D ✗ Suggests biliary obstruction
  E ✗ None proven to be effective

4.40 A ✗ Indicated if serum bilirubin >100 mmol/L
  B ✗ But indicated if severe hyponatraemia is not due to diuretic therapy
  C ✔ Also if ascites is resistant to medical therapy
  D ✗ But hypoxaemia may be due to pulmonary shunting (hepato-pulmonary syndrome)
  E ✗ Contraindicated due to poor prognosis ONLY if hepatoma >5 cm or if multiple

4.41 A ✗ Common hepatic duct
  B ✗ Normal common bile duct <8 mm in diameter
  C ✗ Distal common bile duct usually joins pancreatic duct
  D ✗ Principally vagal tone controls the gallbladder muscle wall
  E ✔

4.42 A ✘ Commoner in North America, Europe and Australia
B ✘ 40% of patients >60 years old
C ✘ Cholesterol stones (pigment stones are more common in developing countries)
D ✔ Usually calcium bilirubinate
E ✘ Hepatic hypersecretion of cholesterol more important

4.43 A ✘ Cystic duct or gallbladder neck is obstructed in 90%
B ✘ 50% are infected
C ✘ May be acalculous
D ✘ Even though intrabiliary pressure may rise
E ✔ Most gallstones are not visible on plain X-ray (radiolucent not radio-opaque)

4.44 A ✘ Associated with gallstones and ulcerative colitis
B ✔ Often with weight loss
C ✘ Suggests hepatocellular carcinoma
D ✘ Often more than 2.5 times normal but non-specific finding
E ✘ Commonest treatment is palliative stenting

4.45 A ✘ Female preponderance—most aged >70 years
B ✘ Adenocarcinoma
C ✔ Gallbladder calcification is common and the disease may be first apparent on USS
D ✘ Such a finding suggests ovarian carcinoma
E ✘ Often advanced at diagnosis since presentation is usually late

5

Clinical haematology and oncology

QUESTIONS

5.1 **Which ONE of the following statements about the normal formation of blood cells is TRUE?**
A   Haematopoiesis is apparent in the bone marrow from the fifth month in utero
B   B lymphocytes but not T lymphocytes originate in the bone marrow
C   Haematopoiesis in adults ceases to occur in the femora and humeri heads
D   The normoblast precedes the development of the proerythroblast
E   Erythropoietin is produced by the Ito cells in the liver

5.2 **Which ONE of the following statements about mature erythrocytes is TRUE?**
A   RBCs express blood group antigens only in the red cell membrane
B   RBCs stain with methylene blue due to ribosomal production of haemoglobin
C   RBCs derive energy from triglycerides to fuel the Na^+/K^+ ionic pump
D   RBCs have a circulation half-life of about 20 days
E   RBCs contain decarboxylase to mediate carbon dioxide transport

5.3 **Which ONE of the following statements about normal haemoglobin is TRUE?**
A   Hb F comprises two alpha and two delta chains
B   Hb A_2 comprises two alpha and two gamma chains
C   Hb has five porphyrin rings each containing ferrous iron
D   Hb is an important buffer of carbonic acid
E   The oxygen binding of Hb is increased by 2–3-diphosphoglycerate within the red cells

5.4 **Which ONE of the following statements about mature neutrophil leucocytes (WBCs) is TRUE?**
A   Neutrophils typically comprise 33% of the total peripheral blood white blood cells in adults
B   Neutrophils remain in the circulation for about 48 hours
C   Neutrophils exhibit increased nuclear segmentation in infection
D   Neutrophils are derived from a different progenitor cell to that of monocytes
E   Neutrophils produce the vitamin B_{12} binding protein transcobalamin III

5.5 **Which ONE of the following statements about white blood cells is TRUE?**
A   Neutrophils are phagocytic and are involved in the killing of protozoa and helminths
B   Basophils bind IgM antibody on their surface and are involved in hypersensitivity reactions
C   Monocytes migrate into the tissues to become T lymphocytes
D   B lymphocytes mediate cellular immunity
E   T lymphocytes comprise CD4 positive helper cells and CD8 positive suppressor cells

5.6 **Which ONE of the following changes in the peripheral blood leucocyte count is associated with the disorders listed below?**
A   Eosinopenia — malaria
B   Neutropenia — Cushing's syndrome
C   Basophilia — hyperthyroidism
D   Lymphopenia — renal failure
E   Basopenia — myeloproliferative disorders

5.7 **Which ONE of the following statements about iron metabolism is TRUE?**
A   The iron content of blood is about 50 micrograms per litre
B   Iron loss in the healthy male is about 3 mg per day
C   The iron content of the adult body is about 5 g
D   Iron is usually stored in hepatocytes as haemosiderin
E   The iron content of a healthy diet is about 1–2 mg per day

5.8 **A 45-year-old woman consults her general practitioner with lethargy and shortness of breath. A full blood count revealed a haemoglobin 54 g/L, MCV 104 fL and reticulocyte count 10% with a normal platelet count but increased white cell count. The plasma haptoglobin concentration was reduced and the direct Coomb's test is positive. Which ONE of the following diagnoses best explains the findings?**
A   Bacterial endocarditis associated with a prosthetic heart valve
B   Mycoplasmal pneumonia
C   Megaloblastic anaemia
D   Malarial infection
E   Chronic lymphatic leukaemia

5.9 **Which ONE of the following features is MOST characteristic of myelofibrosis?**
A   Absence of splenomegaly
B   Leucoerythroblastic blood film with teardrop poikilocytes
C   Decreased leucocyte neutrophil alkaline phosphatase score
D   Hypouricaemia
E   Absence of bone marrow megakaryocytes

5.10 **A 78-year-old presents with confusion and is found to have a raised serum calcium concentration. Serum protein electrophoresis reveals a monoclonal band in the gamma globulin region associated with decreased serum IgM and IgG concentrations. Which ONE of the following suggests a good prognosis?**
A   Serum albumin 22 g/L
B   Decreased serum beta$_2$-microglobulin concentration
C   Blood haemoglobin 70 g/L
D   Bence-Jones protein >500 mg/L
E   Absence of megakaryocytes on bone marrow cytology

5.11 **Which ONE of the following features suggests an alternative diagnosis to Waldenström's macroglobulinaemia?**
A   Hyperviscosity syndrome
B   IgA paraproteinaemia
C   Cryoglobulinaemia
D   Bone marrow infiltration with lymphocytes and mast cells
E   Normal isotope bone scan

5.12 **Which ONE of the following is more likely to produce thrombocytopenic purpura than non-thrombocytopenic purpura?**
A   Waldenström's macroglobulinaemia
B   Henoch–Schönlein purpura
C   Ascorbic acid deficiency
D   Fat embolism
E   Haemolytic-uraemic syndrome

5.13 **Which ONE of the following is more likely to be associated with a haemorrhagic disorder due to deficiency of a clotting factor than a vascular defect?**
A   Von Willebrand's disease
B   Ehlers–Danlos disease
C   Septicaemia
D   Christmas disease
E   Uraemia

5.14 **Which ONE of the following findings suggests an alternative diagnosis to that of disseminated intravascular coagulation?**
A   Thrombocytopenia
B   Schistocytes in the peripheral blood
C   Increased serum fibrin degradation products (FDPs)
D   Normal prothrombin time and thrombin time
E   Increased activated partial thromboplastin time

5.15 Which ONE of the following statements about clotting factors is TRUE?

A Factor V is synthesized by platelets but not by endothelial cells

B Factors V and XII are both activated by carboxylation of their glutamate residues

C Protein C and protein S interact to produce inhibition of factors VIII and IX

D Heparin enhances the inhibitory action of antithrombin on factor Xa and thrombin

E Warfarin acts by inhibition of vitamin K dehydrogenase

5.16 Which ONE of the following facts about the primary antiphospholipid antibody syndrome is TRUE?

A Antibodies impair factor VIII receptor activity

B An increased prevalence in venous but not arterial thromboses is characteristic

C Confirmation of the disorder is provided by the Russell viper venom test

D Tests for cardiolipin antibodies and/or lupus anticoagulant are usually negative

E A peripheral blood thrombocytosis is a typical finding

5.17 Which ONE of the following groups of patients is better treated with compression stockings than heparin therapy to prevent pulmonary thromboembolism?

A Patients admitted with acute myocardial infarction

B Patients with a previous history of DVT admitted with congestive cardiac failure

C Patients who are about to undergo surgery for abdominal malignancy

D Patients with a previous DVT who are admitted for cataract surgery

E Patients admitted to hospital with an acute stroke

5.18 Which ONE of the following statements about platelets is TRUE?

A Platelets have a circulation lifespan of 10 hours in healthy subjects

B They are produced and regulated under the control of erythropoietin

C They contain small nuclear remnants called Howell–Jolly bodies

D The platelet count decreases in response to aspirin therapy

E Platelets release serotonin and von Willebrand factor (vWF)

5.19 A 70-year-old man presents with breathlessness and appears anaemic. The haemoglobin is reduced at 67 g/L. Which ONE of the following peripheral blood findings suggests iron deficiency?
A Macrocytosis
B Ovalocytosis
C Normal mean corpuscular haemoglobin concentration
D Presence of Howell–Jolly bodies
E Thrombocytopenia

5.20 A 35-year-old woman presents with menorrhagia and tiredness. Blood tests confirm anaemia, haemoglobin 91 g/L, MCV 69 fL and the blood film shows hypochromia. Which ONE of the following statements about her management with oral iron therapy is TRUE?
A Folic acid should also be given if the anaemia is severe
B Treatment should be stopped as soon as haemoglobin normalizes
C The haemoglobin should rise by 10 g/L every 7–10 days
D The maximal reticulocyte count usually develops within 1–2 days
E Parenteral iron therapy is likely to be more effective than oral iron therapy

5.21 In a 48-year-old man presenting with tiredness, the full blood count reveals a haemoglobin 97 g/L, MCV 108 fL, platelets 108×10^9/L and white cell count 2.8 10^6/L with hypersegmentation of the nuclei. Which ONE of the following disorders is LEAST likely to explain the blood findings?
A Folic acid deficiency
B Haemolytic anaemia
C Alcohol abuse
D Primary sideroblastic anaemia
E Myelodysplastic syndrome

5.22 A 60-year-old woman presents with weight loss and pallor and is found to have a megaloblastic anaemia Which ONE of the following features would suggest that the disorder is due to vitamin B_{12} deficiency rather than folic acid deficiency?
A Weakness of the lower limbs
B Glossitis
C Splenomegaly
D Peripheral neuropathy
E Diarrhoea

5.23 Which ONE of the following features would suggest an alternative diagnosis to that of a myelodysplastic syndrome?
A Presentation before the age of 30 years
B Macrocytic anaemia and pancytopenia
C Ring sideroblasts present on bone marrow cytology
D Chromosomal abnormalities on cytogenetic analysis
E Subsequent progression to an acute leukaemia

5.24   **Which ONE of the following features is MOST consistent with the diagnosis of primary aplastic anaemia?**
A   Peak incidence about the age of 60 years
B   Normocytic normochromic anaemia with thrombocytosis
C   Pathognomonic changes on the peripheral blood film
D   Palpable splenomegaly
E   Pancytopenia

5.25   **Which ONE of the following features is characteristic of intravascular haemolysis?**
A   Bilirubinuria and haemoglobinuria
B   Absence of methaemalbuminaemia or haemosiderinuria
C   Increased serum haptoglobin concentration
D   Decreased plasma haemoglobin concentration
E   Rigors and persistent fever

5.26   **Which ONE of the following features is characteristic of hereditary spherocytosis?**
A   Absence of splenomegaly
B   Intravascular haemolysis
C   Decreased RBC osmotic fragility
D   Transient aplastic anaemia
E   Increased red cell spectrin concentration

5.27   **Which ONE of the following is the MOST typical feature of adult sickle-cell disease?**
A   Aplastic anaemia
B   Neonatal spherocytic haemolytic anaemia
C   Pulmonary emphysema
D   Splenomegaly with hypersplenism
E   Polyarthritis

5.28   **Which ONE of the following is the MOST typical feature of beta-thalassaemia major?**
A   Macrocytic anaemia
B   Absence of hepatosplenomegaly
C   Absence of pigment gallstones
D   Neonatal haemolytic anaemia
E   Chronic leg ulceration

5.29   **A 79-year-old woman presents with mild jaundice and anaemia. Urinalysis shows no evidence of bilirubinaemia. Which ONE of the following features suggests an alternative diagnosis to that of an autoimmune haemolytic anaemia?**
A   Peripheral blood spherocytosis and splenomegaly
B   Fever with haemoglobinuria and haemosiderinuria
C   Increased serum haptoglobin concentration
D   Positive Coomb's test
E   Previous history of chronic lymphatic leukaemia

5.30 **Which ONE of the following features is the MOST useful in distinguishing polycythaemia rubra vera from secondary causes of polycythaemia?**
A   Increased erythropoiesis in the bone marrow
B   Presence of splenomegaly, leucocytosis and thrombocytosis
C   Absence of symptoms
D   Decreased leucocyte alkaline phosphatase score
E   Decreased blood viscosity

5.31 **Which ONE of the following statements about acute lymphoblastic leukaemia is TRUE?**
A   It has a peak prevalence in patients aged 20–30 years
B   Cytoplasmic Auer rods are typically present in blast cells
C   The median survival with chemotherapy is 30 months
D   It is the commonest of all acute leukaemias
E   It often complicates the late stages of multiple myeloma

5.32 **Which ONE of the following findings in a patient suspected of having chronic myeloid leukaemia suggests an alternative diagnosis?**
A   Painful splenomegaly
B   Sternal tenderness
C   Generalized lymphadenopathy
D   Absence of a bleeding tendency
E   Decreased neutrophil leucocyte alkaline phosphatase score

5.33 **Which ONE of the following findings in a patient suspected of having chronic lymphatic leukaemia suggests an alternative diagnosis?**
A   Onset at the age 65 years
B   Development of autoimmune haemolytic anaemia
C   Massive hepatosplenomegaly at presentation
D   Hypogammaglobulinaemia
E   Mild thrombocytopenia and normal plasma urate

5.34 **In which ONE of the following disorders is allogeneic bone marrow transplantation (BMT) LEAST likely to be of proven benefit?**
A   Multiple myeloma
B   Graft-versus-host disease
C   Alpha-thalassaemia
D   Severe combined immunodeficiency disorder
E   Acute leukaemia

5.35 **In which ONE of the following disorders would the presence of lymphadenopathy and splenomegaly suggest an alternative or additional diagnosis?**
A   Acute lymphoblastic leukaemia
B   Chronic lymphatic leukaemia
C   Hodgkin's lymphoma
D   Non-Hogkin's lymphoma
E   Hairy cell leukaemia

5.36 **Which ONE of the following features in a patient with myelofibrosis suggests an alternative or additional diagnosis?**
A Presence of splenomegaly
B Leucoerythroblastic blood film with teardrop poikilocytes
C Increased leucocyte neutrophil alkaline phosphatase score
D Folic acid deficiency and hyperuricaemia
E Absent bone marrow megakaryocytes and thrombocytopenia

5.37 **Which ONE of the following features in a patient with multiple myeloma suggests an alternative or additional diagnosis?**
A Onset at age 29 years
B Presence of amyloidosis
C Median survival of about 10 years with chemotherapy
D Recurrent infections and pancytopenia
E Increased serum calcium, urate and blood urea

5.38 **In differentiating multiple myeloma from benign monoclonal gammopathy, which ONE of the following findings MOST supports a diagnosis of multiple myeloma?**
A The presence of a monoclonal gammopathy with normal serum immunoglobulin levels
B Bone marrow plasma cell count 5%
C Bilateral carpal tunnel syndrome
D Absence of Bence-Jones proteinuria
E Normal isotope bone scan

5.39 **Which ONE of the following histopathological findings is the MOST typical feature of Hodgkin's disease?**
A Presence of Reed–Sternberg binucleate giant cells
B Decreased tissue eosinophils, neutrophils and plasma cells
C Decreased fibrous stroma in the nodular sclerosing type
D Frequent involvement of the central nervous system
E Absence of histopathological changes in the spleen

5.40 **Which ONE of the following coagulation defects typically produces a prolongation of the prothrombin time?**
A Defects of the intrinsic pathway
B Factor XI deficiency
C Factor VII deficiency
D Factor VI deficiency
E Factor XII deficiency

5.41 **The activated partial thromboplastin time (APTT) is typically prolonged in which ONE of the following coagulation defects?**
A Disorders of the extrinsic pathway
B Factor VII deficiency
C Factor VIII deficiency
D Factor XIII deficiency
E Factor VI deficiency

5.42 **Which ONE of the following statements about von Willebrand disease is TRUE?**
A   The disorder is inherited in an X-linked recessive mode
B   It is characterized by a prolonged prothrombin time
C   The von Willebrand factor (vWF) is synthesized by tissue macrophages
D   The vWF is bound to factor VIII and forms bridges between platelets and endothelial cells
E   Deficiency of vWF is best treated by somatostatin therapy

5.43 **A 35-year-old man presents with excessive bleeding around the socket of a recently extracted tooth. There is no family history as the patient was adopted. Clinical examination showed no evidence of bruising or petechiae. Which ONE of the following findings would support a diagnosis of mild haemophilia A?**
A   History of recurrent haemarthroses in childhood
B   Platelet count 80×10^9L
C   Bleeding time 5 minutes
D   Prothrombin ratio 1.9
E   Prolonged activated partial thromboplastin time at 120 sec

5.44 **Which ONE of the following features is LEAST likely to result from a blood transfusion reaction?**
A   Urticaria
B   Congestive cardiac failure
C   Development of Rhesus antibodies in a Rhesus-negative patient
D   Hypercalcaemia
E   Acute intravascular haemolysis

5.45 **A 60-year-old man receives a blood transfusion following radical prostatectomy and later becomes acutely unwell. Which ONE of the following features suggests that the diagnosis cannot be attributed to an acute haemolytic transfusion reaction?**
A   Clinical deterioration within minutes of starting the blood transfusion
B   The onset of rigors
C   Severe backache
D   Sudden loss of consciousness
E   Profound hypotension

ANSWERS

5.1   A ✔
      B ✘ All originate in the bone marrow but some migrate to the thymus
      C ✘ From birth most of the bone marrow is haemopoietically active
      D ✘ Proerythroblast is earliest identifiable red cell precursor
      E ✘ Produced by renal cortical fibroblast-like cells

5.2   A ✔
      B ✘ True only of reticulocyte
      C ✘ Glucose is the energy source required to maintain biconcave morphology
      D ✘ 120 days; shorter survival times can be measured using chromium labelling
      E ✘ Carbonic anhydrase converts CO_2 and H_2O to carbonic acid which then dissociates

5.3   A ✘ Two alpha and two gamma
      B ✘ Two alpha and two delta
      C ✘ Four porphyrin rings, methaemoglobin contains a ferric ion
      D ✔ H^+ generated in dissociation buffered by deoxyhaemoglobin
      E ✘ Decreased by RBC 2-3-diphosphoglycerate

5.4   A ✘ Ranges from 40% to 70%; under the age of 7 years, lymphocytes predominate
      B ✘ Survive about 8 hours in the circulation
      C ✘ Decreased nuclear segmentation — a shift to the left in the Arneth count
      D ✘ Both arise from granulocyte-macrophage colony-forming cells
      E ✔ Hence high serum vitamin B_{12} levels in chronic myeloid leukaemia

5.5   A ✘ Eosinophils; they produce peroxidases to generate reactive oxygen
      B ✘ Bind IgE and resemble tissue mast cells
      C ✘ Monocytes transform to tissue macrophages; long-lived phagocytic cells
      D ✘ B lymphocytes (20% of all lymphocytes) mediate humoral immunity
      E ✔

5.6 A ✗ Neutropenia; also occurs in viral infections and salmonellosis

       B ✗ Neutrophilia and eosinopenia; effects of excess corticosteroids and catecholamines

       C ✗ Decreased basophil count

       D ✔ Also in lymphoma and systemic lupus erythematosus

       E ✗ Basophilia; also occurs in iron deficiency

5.7 A ✗ Blood contains 500 mg iron per litre; average menstrual loss is 30 mg per month

       B ✗ Males lose 1 mg per day, females lose 2 mg per day

       C ✔ 60–70% resides in the haemoglobin molecule

       D ✗ Stored as ferritin

       E ✗ 10–15 mg per day of which about 15% is absorbed

5.8 A ✗ But may produce a mechanical intravascular haemolysis

       B ✗ But often associated with cold agglutinins and haemolysis

       C ✗ Low-grade haemolysis

       D ✗ Severe in blackwater fever

       E ✔ Often Coomb's positive AIHA

5.9 A ✗ Massive splenomegaly can occur

       B ✔ Characteristic finding

       C ✗ Increased LAP score; decreased in chronic myeloid leukaemia

       D ✗ Hyperuricaemia due to increased cell turnover

       E ✗ Excess megakaryocytes

5.10 A ✗ Severe hypoalbuminaemia is a feature of advanced myeloma

       B ✔ Prognosis is worse as levels become elevated

       C ✗ Prognosis is also poor if there is renal failure

       D ✗ Rapidly progressive multiple myeloma

       E ✗ Poor prognosis

5.11 A ✗ Haemorrhagic tendency with nosebleeds and bruising

       B ✔ IgM paraproteinaemia

       C ✗ Cryoglobulinaemia occurs in 30% of patients

       D ✗ Characteristic

       E ✗ Like myeloma, bone changes are not detectable on bone scan

5.12 A ✗ Usually associated with hyperviscosity syndrome

       B ✗

       C ✗ Vitamin C deficiency — scurvy

       D ✗

       E ✔ Thrombotic thrombocytopenic purpura (DIC)

5.13 A ✗ Failure to synthesize von Willebrand factor
B ✗ Impaired collagen synthesis impairs capillary support
C ✗ Endothelial damage
D ✔ Factor IX deficiency
E ✗ Platelet dysfunction may also occur in severe hepatic failure

5.14 A ✗ Microangiopathic platelet destruction
B ✗ These red cell fragments may be absent in mild cases
C ✗ Increased FDPs and increased levels of D-dimer
D ✔ Both are prolonged due to factor V and fibrinogen deficiency
E ✗ Due to factors V, VIII and fibrinogen deficiency

5.15 A ✗ Synthesized by both platelets and endothelial cells
B ✗ Factors II, VII, IX and X are activated by carboxylation of their glutamate residues
C ✗ Inhibit factor Va and is often first suspected on finding resistance to heparin
D ✔ Hence the effectiveness of low-dose heparin therapy
E ✗ Inhibits epoxide reductase necessary for vitamin K-dependent carboxylase activity

5.16 A ✗ Antibodies interfere with coagulation reactions associated with platelet membranes
B ✗ Both may occur and can affect every organ system
C ✔ Prolongs the APTT due to an in vitro interaction with phospholipids
D ✗ Characteristically one or both are positive
E ✗ Thrombocytopenia is typical; autoimmune haemolytic anaemia may also occur

5.17 A ✗ At risk of DVT and PE
B ✗ High risk of DVT
C ✗ High risk of DVT
D ✗ Minimal risk of recurrent DVT if mobility is unimpaired
E ✔ Use compression stockings; the risk of intracerebral haemorrhage > benefits

5.18 A ✗ 10-day lifespan
B ✗ Thrombopoietins secreted by the megakaryocytes regulate their production
C ✗ Found in red blood cells
D ✗ Main effect is on platelet function
E ✔ Serotonin (delta granules) and vWF and fibrinogen (alpha granules)

5.19 A ✗ Microcytosis is the first sign
B ✔ Sometimes also poikilocytosis
C ✗ Reduced due to microcytosis
D ✗ Suggests hyposplenism
E ✗ Thrombocytosis occurs even in the absence of bleeding

5.20 A ✘ Only if coexistent deficiency demonstrated
B ✘ Continue for 3 months to replenish stores
C ✔ Unless malabsorption, bleeding or poor compliance occur
D ✘ Reticulocyte count response peaks at 7–10 days
E ✘ Oral iron is usually effective unless malabsorption coexists

5.21 A ✘ Megaloblastic anaemia produces a pancytopenia
B ✘ Folate deficiency commonly coexists
C ✘ Macronormoblastosis and folate deficiency
D ✔ Usually a dimorphic blood picture with microcytes and macrocytes
E ✘ Variable red cell morphology

5.22 A ✔ Subacute combined degeneration of the spinal cord in vitamin B$_{12}$ deficiency only
B ✘ But less common in folate deficiency
C ✘ Due to mild haemolysis
D ✘ Occurs in both
E ✘ Occurs in both

5.23 A ✔ Typically elderly patients
C ✘ Usually with hypercellular dysplastic marrow
C ✘ Ring normoblasts with interrupted perinuclear iron ring
D ✘ Occur in 50% of patients, particularly affecting chromosomes 5 and 7
E ✘ Risk is dependent on the precise type of myelodysplastic syndrome

5.24 A ✘ Peak incidence age about 30 years
B ✘ Thrombocytopenia
C ✘ Diagnosis can only be established by bone marrow trephine
D ✘ Splenomegaly is unusual
E ✔ Typical

5.25 A ✘ Bilirubin is unconjugated therefore not found in urine
B ✘ Presence of both indicates intravascular haemolysis
C ✘ Decreased serum haptoglobin
D ✘ Increased plasma Hb (not serum Hb) bound to serum haptoglobin
E ✔ Often with splenomegaly and reticulocytosis

5.26 A ✘ Splenomegaly and pigment gallstones
B ✘ RBC destruction occurs in the spleen
C ✘ Osmotic fragility is increased
D ✔ Often in association with parvovirus infection
E ✘ Deficiency of red cell spectrin, an RBC membrane protein

5.27 A ✔ Often precipitated by viral infection
B ✗ Not until HbF levels fall after the age of 3 months
C ✗ Pulmonary, splenic, renal and mesenteric infarcts causing pain
D ✗ Splenic atrophy and functional hyposplenism
E ✗ Painful bone infarcts may result in *Salmonella osteomyelitis*

5.28 A ✗ Typically hypochromic microcytic anaemia
B ✗ Common in the 'major' (homozygous) form
C ✗ Chronic haemolysis produces pigment gallstones
D ✗ Not until HbF synthesis declines
E ✔ Also occurs in the 'minor' (heterozygous) form

5.29 A ✗ Characteristic
B ✗ Suggesting intravascular haemolysis
C ✔ Decreased serum haptoglobin concentration
D ✗ Warm agglutinins are usually IgG, cold agglutinins are usually IgM
E ✗ Recognized associations also include SLE and lymphoma

5.30 A ✗ Occurs in both
B ✔ And elevated red cell mass
C ✗ But headaches and pruritus are common
D ✗ A feature of chronic myeloid leukaemia
E ✗ Increased blood viscosity and risk of arterial thromboses

5.31 A ✗ Peak incidence in childhood
B ✗ Seen in acute myeloblastic leukaemia
C ✔ AML has a 40% 5-year survival with chemotherapy
D ✗ AML is four times more common than ALL
E ✗ But may complicate myelofibrosis

5.32 A ✗ Splenomegaly occurs in 90%
B ✗ Common finding
C ✔ Most atypical feature
D ✗ Variable platelet dysfunction
E ✗

5.33 A ✗ Peak incidence age 65 years
B ✗ Coomb's positive — typically warm IgG antibody
C ✔ Mild organomegaly only
D ✗ Associated with a paraproteinaemia in 5%
E ✗ Hyperuricaemia and thrombocytosis more likely in CML

5.34 A ✗ Useful in younger patients
B ✔ A complication of BMT
C ✗ Useful in all severe thalassaemias
D ✗
E ✗

5.35　A　✗
　　　B　✗　Mild splenomegaly and generalized lymphadenopathy are common
　　　C　✗　Moderate lymphadenopathy and splenomegaly
　　　D　✗
　　　E　✔　Splenomegaly without lymphadenopathy

5.36　A　✗　Massive splenomegaly can occur
　　　B　✗　A characteristic finding
　　　C　✗　In contrast to CML
　　　D　✗　Due to increased cell turnover
　　　E　✔　An excess of megakaryocytes is a typical feature

5.37　A　✔　Peak prevalence in males aged 60–70 years
　　　B　✗　Amyloidosis occurs in 10%
　　　C　✗　Median survival of 40 months
　　　D　✗　Reduction of normal plasma cells causes immunodeficiency
　　　E　✗　All of which occur and may be asymptomatic

5.38　A　✗　Myloma produces suppression of the other serum immunoglobulins
　　　B　✗　bone marrow plasma cell count >20%
　　　C　✔　Amyloidosis also causes a restrictive cardiomyopathy
　　　D　✗　Serum paraprotein may be undetectable but BJ protein should be present
　　　E　✗　Can be normal in both; bone deposits may not be apparent on bone scan

5.39　A　✔　A pathognomonic hallmark
　　　B　✗　Increased mixed cellularity type, especially in the elderly
　　　C　✗　Increased fibrous tissue occurs in 70% of patients
　　　D　✗　In contrast to non-Hodgkin's lymphoma
　　　E　✗　Usually involved even when the spleen is not enlarged

5.40　A　✗　Defects of the extrinsic pathway
　　　B　✗　Factor X deficiency (the Stuart-Prower factor)
　　　C　✔　The first factor in extrinsic pathway
　　　D　✗　Factor V deficiency also affects the APTT
　　　E　✗　Defect of the intrinsic pathway

5.41　A　✗　Disorders of the intrinsic pathway
　　　B　✗　Detected by the prothrombin time
　　　C　✔　Factor X also influences the prothrombin time
　　　D　✗　Specific assay required to measure
　　　E　✗　Factors IX, XI and XII are the initial factors of the intrinsic system

5.42 A ✗ Autosomal dominant — gene locus on chromosome 12
      B ✗ Characterized by a prolonged bleeding time
      C ✗ Synthesized by both platelets and endothelial cells
      D ✔ And has a plasma half-life = 12 hours
      E ✗ Desmopressin (DDAVP) therapy increases vWF
             concentrations

5.43 A ✗ Suggests severe haemophilia A
      B ✗ Suggests thrombocytopenic cause
      C ✗ Prolonged in factor VIII deficiency; normal BT >8 minutes
      D ✗ Tests extrinsic system; PTR normal in factor VIII deficiency
      E ✔ Tests intrinsic system; normal APTT <40 sec

5.44 A ✗ An allergic reaction
      B ✗ Volume overload
      C ✗ Particularly important in women of child-bearing age
      D ✔ Hypocalcaemia may complicate massive blood transfusion
      E ✗ Major ABO incompatibility is the likeliest cause

5.45 A ✗ But haemolysis may be delayed for 5–7 days
      B ✗ Stop the transfusion immediately
      C ✗ Also chest pain
      D ✔ Unlikely in the absence of other premonitory changes
      E ✗ May be difficult to diagnose in anaesthetized patients

6

Infectious and sexually transmitted diseases

QUESTIONS

6.1 Which ONE of the following infections is transmitted by the route stated below?
A   Meningococcal infection — faecal–oral spread
B   Legionellosis — faecal–oral spread
C   Giardiasis — faecal–oral spread
D   Listeriosis — airborne spread
E   Gonococcal infection — transplacental spread

6.2 Which ONE of these diagnostic techniques is clinically useful in the following infections?
A   Gastric aspirate microscopy — *Entamoeba histolytica*
B   Stool culture — *Pneumocystis carinii*
C   Bone marrow culture — *Streptococcus pneumoniae*
D   Rising titre of IgM antibodies — *Mycobacterium tuberculosis*
E   Complement fixing antibodies — *Histoplasma capsulatum*

6.3 Which ONE of the following factors is a contraindication to active immunization?
A   Atopic disposition
B   HIV infection if live vaccines are required
C   Pregnancy if killed vaccines are required
D   Chronic cardiac or respiratory failure
E   Family history of allergy to vaccines

6.4 In which ONE of the following infections is a live virus usually used for active immunization?
A   Poliomyelitis
B   Pertussis
C   Typhoid fever
D   Hepatitis A
E   Hepatitis B

6.5 In which ONE of the following disorders is there an indication for passive immunization with human immunoglobulin?
A   Hepatitis C
B   Tetanus
C   Influenza A
D   Meningococcaemia
E   Typhoid fever

6.6 A 23-year-old student consults her general practitioner with a history of painless diarrhoea lasting 5 days following her return from a holiday in North Africa. Which ONE of the following statements is TRUE?
A A causative organism is unlikely to be identifiable from a stool culture
B Antibiotic treatment should be instituted after stool culture has been undertaken
C Antidiarrhoeal agents are particularly useful in children
D Ciprofloxacin therapy is of proven prophylactic benefit
E Doxycycline prophylaxis is advisable for all travellers to sub-Saharan Africa

6.7 Which ONE of the following statements about HIV infection is TRUE?
A An RNA retrovirus
B Transmission via drug abusers occurs more often than by sexual transmission in the UK
C There is no involvement of B lymphocytes
D The virus affects suppressor T lymphocytes more than helper T lymphocytes
E The presence of Kaposi's sarcoma indicates a better prognosis

6.8 Which ONE of the following statements about HIV infection is TRUE?
A 80% of vertically transmitted infections are transplacental
B A child born to an infected mother has a 90% chance of acquiring HIV
C Transmission can occur via breast milk
D Risk of fetal transmission is unaffected by pre-partum antiviral agents
E Vertical transmission is the major mode of transmission worldwide

6.9 Following unprotected sexual intercourse 3 weeks' previously, a 19-year-old girl consults her general practitioner for an 'HIV test'. Which ONE of the following statements is TRUE?
A ELISA testing has a high false negative rate
B Seroconversion typically occurs in under 3 weeks
C A full blood count should be undertaken to check the lymphocyte count
D The virus can be readily cultured from saliva
E Serial testing is necessary to confirm infection in some individuals

6.10 In a patient with AIDS, cryptococcal meningitis is
  A   Less likely to be the cause of meningitis than meningococcal infection
  B   Characterized by abrupt onset of the classical features of a bacterial meningitis
  C   Diagnosed by Indian ink stain of cerebrospinal fluid (CSF)
  D   Typically associated with an abnormal cerebral CT scan
  E   Typically associated with a high CSF polymorph count

6.11 *Pneumocystis carinii* infection in an HIV-positive patient is
  A   The commonest cause of respiratory infection in African patients
  B   Characterized by copious sputum production
  C   Characterized by widespread fine pulmonary crackles
  D   More likely to occur when the CD4 count is <200/mm^3
  E   Excluded by the finding of a normal chest X-ray

6.12 A 16-year-old boy consults his general practitioner with a fever and morbiliform rash and a history that his 3-year-old sister has measles. Which ONE of the following statements is TRUE?
  A   Measles infection is due to a DNA myxovirus
  B   Rhinorrhoea and conjunctivitis occur during the recovery phase of the illness
  C   Koplik's spots appear at the same time as the skin rash
  D   The skin rash typically desquamates as it disappears
  E   The infectivity of measles is confined to the prodromal phase

6.13 Which ONE of the following features is typical of mumps?
  A   Infection with a DNA myxovirus
  B   High infectivity for 3 weeks after the onset of parotitis
  C   Development of an acute lymphocytic meningitis
  D   Abdominal pain is usually attributable to mesenteric adenitis
  E   Orchitis is usually bilateral and predominantly occurs prepubertally

6.14 Which ONE of the following features is typical of rabies?
  A   An enterovirus infection
  B   An incubation period of 4–8 days
  C   A good prognosis if symptoms develop slowly
  D   Encephalitis or ascending paralysis
  E   Active and passive vaccination are useful in prevention and therapy

6.15 Which ONE of the following statements about *Helicobacter pylori* (HP) infection is TRUE?

A The diagnosis can be confirmed by decreased urease concentrations in the gastric mucosa

B The presence of oesophagitis indicates the need for HP eradication therapy

C HP eradication is enhanced by low gastric pH

D Amoxicillin plus metronidazole therapy is more effective than amoxicillin alone

E HP eradication reduces recurrence rates of duodenal ulcers but not gastric ulcers

6.16 A middle-aged woman is referred to hospital with a fever, abdominal pain and diarrhoea. Which ONE of the following statements about *Yersinia* infection is TRUE?

A Transmission of the infection is waterborne

B There is an association with exudative pharyngitis and enterocolitis

C There is an association with chronic ileitis

D Erythema marginatum is a characteristic occurrence

E There is likely to be a good clinical response to benzylpenicillin therapy

6.17 Which ONE of the following clinical features is typical of Lassa fever?

A Endemic infection in South America

B Transmission via the mosquito

C No useful response to any antiviral agent

D Acute liver failure is a recognized complication

E An incubation period of 3–6 weeks

6.18 Which ONE of the following features is typical of yellow fever?

A A togavirus infection transmitted by mosquitoes

B An incubation period of 3–6 weeks

C Peripheral blood leucocytosis in contrast to viral hepatitis

D Fever, headache and severe myalgia with bone pains

E Response to ribavirin drug therapy

6.19 Which ONE of the following is characteristic of an influenza virus infection?

A Occurs exclusively in humans

B Low levels of antigenic shift

C Transmissible by oro–faecal route

D An incubation period of 5–7 days

E Infection complicated by Reye's syndrome

6.20 **Which ONE of the following features is typical of respiratory syncytial virus infection?**
A   Infection is more common in adults than children
B   Infection is best diagnosed by serology
C   Infants are protected from infection due to maternally acquired antibodies
D   Infection is typically associated with bronchiolitis
E   Involvement of the lower urinary tract is characteristic

6.21 **A young man is admitted with right-sided abdominal pain and jaundice. Which ONE of the following features is most consistent with a diagnosis of leptospirosis?**
A   Incubation period of 1–2 months
B   History of leisure pursuits involving inland waterways
C   Absence of fever or constitutional symptoms
D   Development of meningitis suggests infection with *Leptospira icterohaemorrhagiae*
E   Gram-positive rods seen on the blood film

6.22 **Which ONE of the following statements about syphilis is TRUE?**
A   Infection is usually caused by *Treponema pertenue*
B   Untreated, infectivity is restricted to the first 2 months
C   The distinction between early and late syphilis is made at 2 years
D   The incubation period for primary syphilis is typically 6 months
E   Tertiary syphilis usually develops within the first year after the initial infection

6.23 **A 60-year-old businessman consults his doctor worried he may have contracted syphilis. Which ONE of the following statements about secondary syphilis is TRUE?**
A   Macular rash occurs 6 months after the appearance of a penile ulcer
B   Wart-like papules on the perineum suggest tertiary syphilis
C   Generalized lymphadenopathy and oro–genital mucous ulceration
D   Cerebrospinal fluid cytology is likely to demonstrate a pleocytosis
E   The presence of a soft, early diastolic murmur indicates secondary syphilis

6.24 **In a 28-year-old woman presenting with a vaginal discharge, which ONE of the following features suggests an alternative diagnosis to that of gonorrhoea?**
A   An incubation period of 3–4 weeks
B   Presence of a urethritis
C   Right hypochondrial pain
D   A pustular haemorrhagic rash
E   An acute monoarthritis of the knee joint

6.25 Which ONE of the following statements about bacteraemic shock is TRUE?
A Endotoxin initiates disseminated intravascular coagulation
B Peripheral vascular resistance remains normal throughout
C Acute circulatory failure is usually due to cardiac failure
D Leucocytosis and thrombocythaemia indicate a poor prognosis
E Antibiotic therapy should await bacteriological results

6.26 In a patient presenting with a sore throat, diphtheria rather than streptococcal tonsillitis is suggested by which ONE of the following findings?
A Tender cervical lymphadenopathy
B Bloodstained nasal discharge
C A tonsillar exudate that is easily removed with a spatula
D Normal movement of the soft palate
E Onset with a high fever and rigors

6.27 A farm worker presents with a fever following laceration of his left shin. Which ONE of the following features most suggests the development of tetanus?
A An incubation period of 2–3 days
B Muscular spasm typically starting in the masseters
C Convulsions associated with loss of consciousness
D Absence of abdominal muscle rigidity
E Bacteriological isolation of *Clostridium tetani* from the wound

6.28 Which ONE of the following statements about the treatment of tetanus is TRUE?
A Tetanus toxoid should be given intravenously as soon as possible
B Wound debridement should be undertaken prior to any other therapy
C Human antitetanus immunoglobulin should be given immediately
D Diazepam should be avoided because of the hazards of oversedation
E Cephalosporin therapy is the antibiotic treatment of choice

6.29 Following a meal at a local restaurant, a 31-year-old woman is admitted with collapse. Which ONE of the following features MOST suggests botulism?
A Ingestion of infected material 2–4 hours prior to the onset of symptoms
B Onset with an acute gastroenteritis associated with postural hypotension
C Absence of autonomic nervous system involvement
D Bulbar palsy developing slowly over 10–14 days
E Dramatic clinical response to parenteral antitoxin

6.30 Which ONE of the following features is typical of anthrax?
A   Occupational exposure to fish products
B   An incubation period of 1–3 weeks
C   Painful lymphadenopathy
D   Presentation with bronchopneumonia
E   Multiple antibiotic resistance is common

6.31 Which ONE of the following features is characteristic of leprosy?
A   An incubation period of 3–6 weeks
B   Growth of the organism on Lowenstein–Jensen medium after 2–3 months
C   Spread of the tuberculoid form on prolonged patient contact
D   Spontaneous healing of the earliest macule
E   A cell-mediated immune response in the lepromatous form

6.32 Which ONE of the following features is characteristic of lepromatous leprosy?
A   Absence of infectivity of affected patients
B   Unlike the tuberculoid form, organisms are scanty in number
C   Blood-borne spread from the dermis throughout the body
D   Strongly positive lepromin skin test
E   Anaesthetic hypopigmented skin macules and plaques

6.33 Which ONE of the following statements about the life cycle of plasmodia is TRUE?
A   Sporozoites disappear from the blood 3–7 days post-infection
B   Merozoites re-entering red blood cells undergo sexual but not asexual reproduction
C   All plasmodia multiply in the liver but not in the red blood cells
D   Dormant hypnozoites remain within the liver cells in all species
E   Fertilization of the gametocytes occurs in the human red blood cells

6.34 Which ONE of the following statements about the diagnosis and therapy of amoebiasis is TRUE?
A   The presence of cystic forms of amoeba can be demonstrated in most amoebic liver abscesses
B   Stool trophozoites are unlikely to be found in the rectal mucus
C   Liver abscesses are often undetected by liver ultrasound scanning
D   Metronidazole therapy is effective in both liver and colonic disease
E   Diloxanide therapy is ineffective in eliminating amoebic cysts in the colon

6.35 **Which ONE of the following statements about visceral leishmaniasis is TRUE?**
   A Spread of *Leishmania donovani* is principally via anopheline mosquitoes
   B An incubation period of 1–2 weeks
   C Rigors with hepatomegaly but no splenomegaly is a typical clinical feature
   D Diagnosis is best confirmed by microscopy of a peripheral blood film
   E A good clinical response to pentavalent antimonial therapy is to be expected

6.36 **Which ONE of the following features is typical of cutaneous leishmaniasis?**
   A Nasal and mouth mucosal ulcers
   B Painful ulcers in the groins or axillae
   C Marked splenomegaly and lymphadenopathy
   D Ulcers which heal without scarring
   E Negative leishmanin skin test

6.37 **Which ONE of the following features is typical of *Schistosoma haematobium* infection?**
   A Disease confined to the urinary tract
   B Presentation with painless haematuria
   C Spontaneous resolution within a year of leaving endemic areas
   D Absence of involvement of the uterine cervix and seminal vesicles
   E An endemic disease in China and the Far East

6.38 **Which ONE of the following statements about coxsackie B virus infection is TRUE?**
   A The virus is an RNA arbor virus
   B It causes hand, foot and mouth disease
   C It is a typical cause of pancreatitis
   D It is a likely cause of aseptic meningitis
   E It is a likely cause of herpangina

6.39 **A 35-year-old man returns from a holiday in Egypt with a fever, headache and severe limb pains. Which ONE of the following features most suggests dengue fever?**
   A History of a rat bite 2 weeks previously
   B Marked peripheral blood leucocytosis
   C Cervical lymphadenopathy
   D Erythema nodosum
   E Yellow fever vaccination prior to travelling

6.40 **Which ONE of the following infections is attributable to chlamydial organisms?**
  A Psittacosis
  B Epidemic typhus
  C Yellow fever
  D Yaws
  E Q fever

6.41 **Which ONE of the following statements about trachoma is TRUE?**
  A Blepharospasm is a common presenting feature
  B It is often complicated by acute glaucoma producing blindness
  C Acute ophthalmia neonatorum is a recognized presentation
  D Treatment with penicillin eye drops is likely to be effective
  E Blindness is usually due to the formation of cataracts

6.42 **A 50-year-old housewife presents with a febrile illness characterized by a cough. Which ONE of the following features is most consistent with the diagnosis of psittacosis?**
  A An incubation period of 4 weeks
  B An acute small joint polyarthritis
  C Pulmonary infiltrates on chest X-ray not apparent on clinical examination
  D The family pet snake was recently unwell and required antibiotic therapy
  E Prompt resolution with sulphonamide therapy

ANSWERS

6.1   A   ✘   Airborne spread
      B   ✘   Water aerosols especially from air-conditioning systems
      C   ✔   As in *Campylobacter* infection
      D   ✘   Via ingestion of cheese, especially in the elderly or immunosuppressed
      E   ✘   But syphilis may be transmitted in maternal blood

6.2   A   ✘   Rectal biopsy and stool microscopy in amoebic dysentery
      B   ✘   Lung biospy and sputum microscopy
      C   ✘   Useful in e.g. brucellosis, tuberculosis
      D   ✘   Useful in brucella and other infections
      E   ✔

6.3   A   ✘
      B   ✔   Also contraindicated in other immunosuppressed states
      C   ✘
      D   ✘
      E   ✘

6.4   A   ✔   Inactivated vaccine also available
      B   ✘
      C   ✘
      D   ✘
      E   ✘

6.5   A   ✘   Unlike hepatitis A and B
      B   ✔   For susceptible injured patients
      C   ✘
      D   ✘
      E   ✘

6.6   A   ✘   Common causes include *Escherichia coli*
      B   ✘   Most resolve spontaneously
      C   ✘   Avoid, may cause toxic dilatation of the bowel
      D   ✔
      E   ✘   Reserve for susceptible individuals

6.7   A   ✔
      B   ✘   Promiscuity and male homosexuality are common risk factors in the UK
      C   ✘   Greater effect on T lymphocytes
      D   ✘   CD4 helper T cells are principally involved
      E   ✘   Prognosis is worse with Kaposi's sarcoma

6.8   A   ✘   Majority occur during parturition
      B   ✘   Under 50% chance
      C   ✔   10–20% additional risk for breastfed babies
      D   ✘   Zidovudine can reduce transmission rate
      E   ✘   Heterosexual transmission is the major mode worldwide (75%)

6.9   A   ✗   Low false negative rate and used as an effective screening test
       B   ✗   6–12 weeks or longer
       C   ✗   Lymphopenia is a feature of AIDS
       D   ✗   Cultured from peripheral blood lymphocytes
       E   ✔   Because of delay in seroconversion in some patients

6.10   A   ✗   The commonest cause of meningitis and also causes pulmonary disease
       B   ✗   Poor inflammatory response masks classical features
       C   ✔   And serum/CSF culture
       D   ✗   Normal cerebral CT scan
       E   ✗   CSF monocytosis is typical

6.11   A   ✗   Tuberculosis is common
       B   ✗   Dry cough and dyspnoea
       C   ✗   Crackles would be unusual
       D   ✔   In 95% of cases
       E   ✗   Normal chest X-ray is found in 10% of cases

6.12   A   ✗   Single-stranded RNA paramyxovirus
       B   ✗   At the onset — the catarrhal phase
       C   ✗   Precede the rash
       D   ✔
       E   ✗   Avoid contact for 7 days after the onset of the rash

6.13   A   ✗   RNA paramyxovirus spread by airborne droplets
       B   ✗   Infectivity is generally low
       C   ✔
       D   ✗   Pain suggests pancreatitis or oophoritis
       E   ✗   It is usually unilateral and postpubertal

6.14   A   ✗   A rhabdovirus infection especially endemic in bats, dogs and foxes
       B   ✗   Average 4–8 weeks
       C   ✗   Usually fatal
       D   ✔
       E   ✗

6.15   A   ✗   Urease levels in the gastric mucosa are increased due to the presence of HP (CLO test)
       B   ✗   HP eradication has no clinically significant effect on oesophagitis
       C   ✗   Hence concomitant acid-lowering drug therapy in eradication regimes
       D   ✔   Eradication rates are increased from 65% to 90% by therapy with these two antibiotics
       E   ✗   Recurrence rates for both are >90% without HP eradication

6.16 A ✗ Zoonoses endemic in pigs, domestic animals and birds
 B ✔
 C ✗ Acute ileitis and mesenteric adenitis especially with
 Y. pseudotuberculosis
 D ✗ Erythema nodosum and reactive arthritis especially with
 Y. enterocolitica
 E ✗ Tetracycline or gentamicin are more useful

6.17 A ✗ Sub-Saharan West Africa
 B ✗ Typically via infected urine or body fluids
 C ✗ Ribavarin may be useful
 D ✔ In severe cases
 E ✗ 3–6 days

6.18 A ✗ A flavivirus enzootic in monkeys and transmitted by
 mosquitoes
 B ✗ 3–6 days
 C ✗ Leucopenia
 D ✔
 E ✗ Supportive therapy only

6.19 A ✗ Infects many other animals
 B ✗ High level of antigenic shift associated with pandemic
 infection
 C ✗ Transmissible by respiratory secretions
 D ✗ 1–3 days
 E ✔ Occurs in children given aspirin therapy

6.20 A ✗ Major cause of lower respiratory tract infection in children
 B ✗ Immunofluorescence of throat swabs may be useful
 C ✗ Offers no protection
 D ✔ Also pneumonia
 E ✗ Cough is usually the dominant feature

6.21 A ✗ 7–14 days
 B ✔ Also abattoirs and farms
 C ✗ Severe myalgia, headache and conjunctival suffusion
 D ✗ *L. canicola* infection usually presents as aseptic meningitis
 E ✗ Spirochaete-like organisms seen on the blood film suggest
 Borrelia or *Leptospira* organisms

6.22 A ✗ Due to infection with *Treponema pallidum*
 B ✗ Infectivity persists if untreated
 C ✔
 D ✗ 14–28 days but may be up to 90 days
 E ✗ Takes at least 2 years to develop

6.23 A ✘ Fever and a macular rash occur 8 weeks after the chancre, often with lymphadenopathy
B ✘ Condylomata lata are characteristic of secondary syphilis
C ✔ 'Snail-track' ulcers
D ✘ Meningeal involvement is rare
E ✘ Cardiac involvement is a feature of tertiary disease

6.24 A ✔ Usually 2–10 days
B ✘ Dysuria is more common in males than females, discharge or no symptoms
C ✘ Due to perihepatitis from trans-peritoneal spread (Fitz-Hugh–Curtis syndrome)
D ✘ Associated with gonococcal septicaemia (affects females especially)
E ✘ Septic arthritis

6.25 A ✔
B ✘ Often falls initially due to vasodilatation before rising
C ✘ Due to peripheral vasodilation and capillary damage
D ✘ Leucopenia suggests a poorer prognosis
E ✘ Urgent antibiotic therapy after taking the appropriate cultures

6.26 A ✘ May occur in either
B ✔ Suggests anterior nasal infection and myocarditis
C ✘ Streptococcal exudate is easily removed
D ✘ Paralysis of the soft palate and/or ocular muscles
E ✘ Typical of streptococcal tonsillitis

6.27 A ✘ May be as long as several weeks
B ✔ Causing trismus
C ✘ Painful muscle contractions
D ✘ Abdominal rigidity without pain or tenderness
E ✘ Not often achieved

6.28 A ✘ Antitoxin is given intravenously
B ✘ Antitoxin should be given as soon as possible
C ✔
D ✘ Necessary to control spasms
E ✘ Penicillin therapy or if allergic, metronidazole therapy

6.29 A ✘ 12–72 hours after ingestion
B ✔
C ✘ Autonomic neuropathy induced by the cholinergic neurotoxin
D ✘ Diplopia and bulbar palsy may occur within 1–3 days
E ✘ Tissue-bound toxin cannot be neutralized

6.30 A ✗ Exposure to animals and animal products, e.g. farmers, butchers and those dealing with wool, hides and bone meal
  B ✗ 1–3 days
  C ✗ Painless skin nodule with regional lymphadenopathy
  D ✔ Also gastroenteritis and meningitis
  E ✗ Organism is widely chemosensitive

6.31 A ✗ 3–6 years
  B ✗ Organism cannot be grown in artificial media
  C ✗ No risk of infection in tuberculoid leprosy
  D ✔
  E ✗ Characteristic of the tuberculoid form

6.32 A ✗ Infectivity is high
  B ✗ Is multi-bacillary disease
  C ✔ No cell-mediated immune response
  D ✗ Suggests tuberculoid disease
  E ✗ Macules occur, but sensation is retained

6.33 A ✔ Sporozoites enter the liver within 30 minutes of innoculation
  B ✗ Both sexual and asexual reproduction
  C ✗ Merozoites enter the RBCs and multiply asexually
  D ✗ Only *P. vivax* and *P. ovale* persist in this form
  E ✗ Fertilization occurs in the mosquito

6.34 A ✗ Free amoebae or cysts are rarely found
  B ✗ Exudate in the stool should be examined for trophozoites
  C ✗ Ultrasound-guided aspiration is useful
  D ✔ Or tinidazole, together with diloxanide therapy
  E ✗ Diloxanide therapy should also be given to eliminate colonic amoebic cysts

6.35 A ✗ By sandflies from dogs and rodents; also from infected blood transfusions
  B ✗ 1 month to 10 years
  C ✗ Splenomegaly is characteristic
  D ✗ Diagnosis by examination of stained smears of bone marrow, spleen or liver
  E ✔ Pentamidine is an effective alternative

6.36 A ✔ Secondary to initial cutaneous ulceration
  B ✗ Typically painless and not involving nodes
  C ✗ This occurs in visceral leishmaniasis
  D ✗
  E ✗ Typically positive except in diffuse cutaneous leishmaniasis

6.37 A ✗ Pulmonary disease also occurs
   B ✓ Due to early egg deposition in the bladder mucosa
   C ✗ Adult worms can live for 20 years
   D ✗
   E ✗ *S. japonicum* is prevalent in this area

6.38 A ✗ An RNA enterovirus of which there are at least 30 strains
   B ✗ Caused by coxsackie A with vesicular rash especially in children
   C ✗ Pleuritis in Bornholm's disease
   D ✓ Together with echoviruses cause 90% of cases of aseptic meningitis
   E ✗ Caused by coxsackie A producing a vesicular eruption of the soft palate

6.39 A ✗ Mosquito-borne infection with an incubation period of 5–6 days
   B ✗ Leucopenia and even thrombocytopenia
   C ✓
   D ✗ A morbilliform rash that starts peripherally
   E ✗ No vaccine is available to protect from dengue

6.40 A ✓ *Chlamydia psittaci*
   B ✗ *Rickettsia prowakezi*
   C ✗ An arbor virus infection
   D ✗ Treponemal spirochaete infection
   E ✗ *Coxiella burnetii*

6.41 A ✗ There may be no symptoms before vision fails
   B ✗ Follicular conjunctivitis of the eyelids is typical with entropion and trichiasis
   C ✓
   D ✗ Topical or oral tetracycline is effective
   E ✗ Blindness is due to corneal scarring

6.42 A ✗ Incubation period 4–14 days
   B ✗ A reactive arthritis is unlikely to occur
   C ✓ As in other 'atypical' pneumonias
   D ✗ Infection of birds; birds surviving the disease may still be highly infectious
   E ✗ Tetracycline therapy is effective

7

Endocrinology

QUESTIONS

7.1   An 18-year-old diabetic girl is admitted in a comatose state. Which ONE of the following clinical features suggests the diagnosis of hypoglycaemia rather than diabetic ketoacidosis?
A   Systemic hypotension
B   Extensor plantar responses
C   Air hunger
D   Dry skin
E   Abdominal pain

7.2   Which ONE of the following statements about diabetes mellitus present for over 20 years in a middle-aged individual is TRUE?
A   Retinal neovascularization resolves with better glycaemic control
B   Microaneurysms are only visible with fluorescein angiography
C   Visual symptoms correlate well with the severity of retinal disease
D   Microalbuminuria suggests renal tubular dysfunction
E   The onset of autonomic neuropathy increases risk of sudden death

7.3   Which ONE of the following findings best characterizes the diagnosis of simple obesity?
A   A body mass index 24
B   Decreased plasma insulin concentration
C   Absence of a family history of obesity
D   Decreased cortisol secretion rate
E   A normal basal metabolic rate after correction for total body mass

7.4   In which ONE of the following disorders would the finding of hyperlipidaemia suggest an alternative or additional diagnosis?
A   Chronic renal failure
B   Diabetes mellitus
C   Hyperthyroidism
D   Alcohol abuse
E   Oestrogen hormone replacement therapy

7.5 A 27-year-old woman presents with a confusional state associated with a plasma glucose 2.1 mmol/L. Which ONE of the following diagnoses can be excluded on the basis of the clinical presentation?

A Primary hepatoma
B Alcohol-induced hypoglycaemia
C Hepatic failure
D Starvation
E Pancreatic islet-cell tumour

7.6 In which ONE of the following disorders would the finding of amyloid deposition on subcutaneous fat biopsy suggest an alternative or additional diagnosis?

A Familial Mediterranean fever
B Multiple myeloma
C Type I diabetes mellitus
D Ankylosing spondyloarthritis
E Rheumatoid arthritis

7.7 An asymptomatic 22-year-old man attends his doctor for a medical examination for life insurance purposes. The past history reveals that at the age of 11 years, he was investigated for short stature and found to have growth hormone deficiency. Which ONE of the following statements is TRUE?

A Panhypopituitarism is likely to be present or develop over time
B He is likely to have an undiagnosed craniopharyngioma
C A genetic deficiency of growth hormone releasing factor is likely
D His body mass index is likely to be in the range 17–19
E Detailed questioning is likely to establish a precocious puberty

7.8 Which ONE of the following statements concerning primary pseudohypoparathyroidism is TRUE?

A The condition is associated with defective coupling of adenyl cyclase with renal parathyroid hormone (PTH) receptors
B The serum concentrations are typically low
C Both the serum calcium and serum phosphate levels are reduced
D A family history of short stature or growth retardation is unlikely
E The response to parathyroid hormone is likely to be slow but sustained

7.9 A 29-year-old woman presents to the medical outpatient department with weight loss. While having her blood pressure taken, the patient developed cramp in the muscles of the hand. Blood tests later showed a normal blood urea and electrolytes, but decreased serum calcium and phosphate. Which ONE of the following disorders is the most likely diagnosis?

A Hyperventilation
B Pyloric stenosis
C Primary hypoadrenalism
D Metastatic bone disease
E Gluten enteropathy

7.10 In the treatment of primary adrenocortical insufficiency, which ONE of the following statements is TRUE?

A Oral cortisol acetate is the glucocorticoid of choice
B Fludrocortisone is often unnecessary unless hyperkalaemia occurs
C The dose of cortisol should not be increased without medical advice
D Adrenal crisis requires intravenous crystalloids and hydrocortisone
E The usual daily maintenance therapy is 50 mg cortisol

7.11 A 40-year-old man presents with infertility associated with oligospermia. Which ONE of the following statements is TRUE?

A Decreased plasma FSH concentrations suggest testicular dysfunction
B Testicular biopsy should be undertaken if the testes are undescended
C Testicular sperm production may still be normal
D Gonadotrophin therapy often restores normal fertility
E Low plasma FSH concentrations suggest obstruction of the vas

7.12 A 21-year-old woman presents with infertility and primary amenorrhoea. Investigations show decreased plasma FSH and LH levels. Which ONE of the following disorders is the likeliest diagnosis?

A Thyrotoxicosis
B Turner's syndrome
C Autoimmune ovarian disease
D 5-alpha-reductase deficiency
E Kallman's syndrome

7.13 Which ONE of the following findings if present, suggests an alternative diagnosis to that of Type I multiple endocrine neoplasia syndrome?

A Family history indicating the disorder is an autosomal dominant trait
B The presence of a functioning pituitary adenoma
C An increased plasma calcitonin concentration
D Increased levels of plasma gastrin
E Recurrent spontaneous hypoglycaemia

113

7.14 **Which ONE of the following findings if present, suggests an alternative diagnosis to that of Type II multiple endocrine neoplasia?**
A   Autosomal dominant mode of inheritance
B   Primary hyperparathyroidism
C   High plasma calcitonin concentration
D   A phaeochromocytoma
E   Wilm's nephroblastoma

7.15 **A 25-year-old female presents with a history of episodes of sweating and unexplained postural hypotension. Which ONE of the following features indicates that the cause is likely to be due to an adrenal rather than extra-adrenal phaeochromocytoma?**
A   Raised plasma adrenaline (epinephrine) concentration
B   Paroxysmal hypertension
C   Recurrent renal calculi
D   Troublesome headaches
E   Weight loss and glycosuria

7.16 **Which ONE of the following findings suggests an alternative diagnosis to that of the syndrome of apparent mineralocorticoid excess (AME)?**
A   A low ratio of free urinary cortisol to cortisone
B   Reduced tissue 11-hydroxysteroid dehydrogenase activity
C   Low plasma renin
D   Hypertension
E   Hypokalaemia

7.17 **Which ONE of the following statements about leptin is TRUE?**
A   Leptin is secreted by the hypothalamus
B   It stimulates neuropeptide Y synthesis
C   It acts on cell surface receptors
D   Plasma leptin concentrations are typically reduced in obese people
E   Leptin inhibits alpha-melanocyte stimulating hormone (αMSH)

7.18 **Which ONE of the following plasma hormone concentrations is most likely to be increased in a woman with polycystic ovary syndrome?**
A   Luteinizing hormone
B   Follicle stimulating hormone
C   Thyroid stimulating hormone
D   Adrenocortical trophic hormone
E   Progesterone

7.19 Which ONE of the following plasma hormones is MOST likely to be decreased in a normal 27-year-old woman 30 weeks pregnant?
A Thyroid stimulating hormone
B Free testosterone
C Renin
D Cortisol
E 1,25 dihydroxycholecalciferol

7.20 A 40-year-old man is undergoing investigations with his wife for infertility. His plasma prolactin concentration is found to be markedly increased. Which ONE of the following findings is most INCONSISTENT with a diagnosis of a prolactinoma due to a pituitary microadenoma?
A Galactorrhoea
B Testicular atrophy
C Reduced beard growth
D Increased body mass index
E Impotence

7.21 A young man presents with longstanding nocturnal pain in the back and in the long bones. Blood tests show normal serum calcium and phosphate concentrations but a reduced serum alkaline phosphatase concentration. Which ONE of the following is the most likely diagnosis?
A Paget's disease
B Osteomalacia
C Hypophosphatasia
D Hyperparathyroidism
E Bony metastasis

7.22 Which ONE of the following features occurring in a 37-year-old man with insulin-dependent diabetes mellitus suggests the development of an additional diagnosis rather than a complication of diabetes mellitus?
A pyoderma gangrenosum
B necrobiosis lipoidica diabeticorum
C lipohypertrophy
D moniliasis
E hypoglycaemia

7.23 A 40-year-old man presents with gynaecomastia. Which ONE of the following diagnoses can be excluded as the cause?
A Bronchogenic carcinoma
B Spironolactone therapy
C XYY karyotype
D Digoxin therapy
E Klinefelter's syndrome

7.24 A man of 50 with weight loss and malaise of 6 months' duration has a serum sodium of 120 mmol/L. Which ONE of the following findings supports the diagnosis of inappropriate ADH secretion?

A Urinary osmolality persistently less than 300 mosmol/kg
B Serum potassium 6 mmol/L
C Nocturia and polyuria
D Collapsed right upper lobe on chest X-ray
E Blood urea 40 mmol/L

7.25 A 45-year-old woman has a plasma potassium of 2.5 mmol/L and plasma bicarbonate of 15 mmol/L. Which ONE of the following diagnoses is MOST compatible with these findings?

A Renal tubular acidosis
B Primary aldosteronism
C Acute digoxin poisoning
D Pyloric stenosis
E Chronic respiratory failure

7.26 A middle-aged woman presents with tremor, palpitations and recent heat intolerance. Which ONE of the following statements is TRUE?

A Carbimazole inhibits the uptake of plasma iodide into the thyroid gland
B A retrosternal goitre is a contraindication to radio-iodine therapy
C The diagnosis is confirmed by an elevated total T4
D The eye signs correlate poorly with the degree of thyrotoxicosis
E Propranolol increases peripheral conversion of T4 to T3

7.27 In a 27-year-old woman with weight loss, which ONE of the following features suggests anorexia nervosa rather than chronic hypopituitarism?

A Decreased skin pigmentation
B Amenorrhoea
C Decreased body hair
D A lowered plasma cortisol level
E Normal body fat

7.28 An elderly woman is found to have a TSH level >100 mU/L and a low plasma T_4 concentration. Which ONE of the following features is INCONSISTENT with a diagnosis of primary hypothyroidism?

A Coma
B Cerebellar ataxia
C Intestinal obstruction
D Pericardial effusion
E Increased hepatic cholesterol synthesis

7.29 **Which ONE of the following clinical findings is more consistent with the diagnosis of pseudohypoparathyroidism rather than primary hypoparathyroidism?**
A   Peripheral paraesthesia
B   Abnormal calcification on skull X-ray
C   Dystonia
D   Cataracts
E   Metacarpal abnormalities

7.30 **A 21-year-old young woman presents with an 18 month history of constipation, polyuria and polydipsia without weight loss. Urinalysis showed no abnormality and the urinary osmolality after an overnight fast was 650 mOsm/kg. Which ONE of the following statements is TRUE?**
A   Diabetes mellitus cannot be excluded by urinalysis alone
B   The serum calcium is likely to be elevated
C   A history of excessive chronic analgesic intake is likely
D   A history of erythema nodosum suggests that polyuria may be due to sarcoidosis
E   The most likely diagnosis is compulsive water drinking

7.31 **Which ONE of the following statements about primary hyperparathyroidism is TRUE?**
A   The serum phosphate is characteristically elevated
B   Urinary phosphate excretion is typically reduced
C   Serum calcium rises in response to treatment with thiazide diuretics
D   The prevalence in the community is about 1:100 000
E   In the young patient, surgery is indicated only if symptoms persist

7.32 **A 17-year-old woman is referred with secondary amenorrhoea. Which ONE of the following diagnoses can be excluded on the grounds of the clinical presentation?**
A   Stein–Leventhal syndrome
B   Hyperthyroidism
C   Cushing's disease
D   Acute psychiatric distress
E   Turner's syndrome

7.33 A 60-year-old man is referred with a goitre and a history of waking at night with pain and numbness in both hands. On questioning, he admits to excessive sweating. The plasma TSH was unrecordable and the growth hormone levels did not change during a glucose tolerance test. Which ONE of the following statements is TRUE?

A   The presence of a visual field defect indicates the need for external irradiation

B   The patient is likely to have thyrotoxicosis

C   The serum calcium is likely to be reduced

D   The presence of hypopituitarism is unlikely

E   A pituitary chromophobe adenoma is the likeliest finding

7.34 Which ONE of the following findings in a patient with congenital adrenal hyperplasia suggests that the disorder is associated with a 21-hydroxylase deficiency?

A   Autosomal dominant inheritance

B   The diagnosis is confirmed by elevated plasma cortisol levels

C   On presentation there is usually evidence of excessive pigmentation

D   The condition presents as testicular hypertrophy in males

E   Atrophy of the clitoris is a characteristic feature

7.35 In a 27-year-old woman with weight loss, amenorrhoea and a goitre, which ONE of the following features excludes the diagnosis of primary thyrotoxicosis?

A   An elevated plasma T_4 level but normal plasma TSH level

B   Good response to carbimazole therapy

C   Absence of exophthalmos

D   Presence of thyroid microsomal antibodies

E   Absence of thyroid calcification on X-ray

7.36 Which ONE of the following statements about anorexia nervosa is TRUE?

A   Plasma cortisol levels are likely to be decreased

B   Plasma growth hormone levels are typically decreased

C   The male/female ratio affected is 1:3

D   Plasma gonadotrophins are characteristically normal

E   Plasma TSH levels are typically normal

7.37 In which ONE of the following disorders would impairment of glucose tolerance be an UNEXPECTED feature?

A   Friedreich's ataxia

B   Down's syndrome

C   Klinefelter's syndrome

D   Sippel's syndrome

E   Huntington's chorea

7.38 With which ONE of the following factors would an increase in the plasma vasopressin secretion rate be an UNEXPECTED feature?
A Ethyl alcohol
B Reduction in plasma volume
C Increased plasma osmolality
D An early response to major surgery
E Morphine administration

7.39 A 55-year-old man presents with loss of libido, glycosuria and painful knees. Which ONE of the following features excludes the diagnosis of haemochromatosis?
A Melanin deposits in the skin
B Spontaneous hypoglycaemia
C Testicular atrophy
D Calcification of the symphysis pubis
E HLA A_3 positive

7.40 A 25-year-old woman is admitted with acute abdominal pain and a previous history of numerous admissions with unexplained abdominal pain. Which ONE of the following findings is LEAST likely to support the diagnosis of acute intermittent porphyria?
A A history of severe photosensitivity
B Elevated plasma porphobilinogen (PBG)
C Past history of exacerbation during pregnancy
D Increased urinary levels of delta-amino-laevulinic acid (ALA)
E Past history of seizures

ANSWERS

7.1   A ✗ Volume depletion suggests DKA
       B ✔ Non-specific sign of neuroglycopenia
       C ✗ Suggests metabolic acidosis due to DKA
       D ✗ Dehydration suggests ketoacidosis
       E ✗ An insensitive indicant seen in DKA

7.2   A ✗ Photocoagulation is indicated
       B ✗ Often the first sign of retinopathy detected at ophthalmoscopy
       C ✗ Occur late and regular examination is mandatory
       D ✗ Suggests glomerular dysfunction and indicates microangiopathy
       E ✔ 30–50% mortality over 10 years

7.3   A ✗ BMI 30+ = obesity, morbid obesity = BMI 40+
       B ✗ Hyperinsulinaemia is common
       C ✗ Commonly found but no single gene defect identifiable
       D ✗ Often associated with an increase in cortisol production
       E ✔ BMR is similar to that of lean subjects

7.4   A ✗ Increased triglycerides and very low density lipoprotein (VLDL)
       B ✗ Increased triglycerides and VLDL but decreased HDL
       C ✔ Hypothyroidism increases cholesterol and LDL
       D ✗ Increased triglycerides, VLDL and HDL
       E ✗ Increased triglycerides and HDL

7.5   A ✗ Also occurs in association with haemangiopericytoma
       B ✗ Due to the inhibition of hepatic gluconeogenesis
       C ✗ Also severe renal failure
       D ✔ Never occurs unless associated with alcohol intake
       E ✗ Insulinoma

7.6   A ✗ Reactive (AA) amyloidosis
       B ✗ Primary (AL) amyloidosis
       C ✔
       D ✗ Reactive (AA) amyloidosis
       E ✗ Reactive (AA) amyloidosis

7.7   A ✗ Usually isolated growth hormone secretory failure
       B ✗ Present in only a small minority of patients
       C ✔ Occurs as an isolated abnormality
       D ✗ Most develop mild–moderate obesity with BMI >25
       E ✗ Puberty not affected

7.8　A　✔　Producing tissue resistance to PTH
　　　B　✗　Increased serum PTH in contrast to primary hypoparathyroidism
　　　C　✗　Low serum calcium and high serum phosphate
　　　D　✗　Common and occasionally a history of mental retardation
　　　E　✗　1-alpha hydroxycholecalciferol is the treatment of choice

7.9　A　✗　Respiratory alkalosis reduces only the ionized calcium
　　　B　✗　Metabolic alkalosis reduces the ionized calcium concentration
　　　C　✗　Hypercalcaemia is more likely to occur
　　　D　✗　Hypercalcaemia due to increased osteoclastic activity
　　　E　✔　Vitamin D malabsorption leading to tetany

7.10　A　✗　Oral hydrocortisone; cortisol acetate requires hepatic metabolism
　　　B　✗　Mineralocorticoid is invariably required
　　　C　✗　Patients must increase dose during intercurrent illnesses
　　　D　✔　And consideration of the underlying precipitating cause
　　　E　✗　Usually 30–40 mg per day

7.11　A　✗　Increased plasma FSH occurs following severe orchitis
　　　B　✗　Maldescended testes in an adult should be removed
　　　C　✔　Anti-sperm antibodies may be the cause of oligospermia
　　　D　✗　No treatment is particularly effective
　　　E　✗　Suggests a pituitary or hypothalamic cause

7.12　A　✗　High plasma FSH and LH
　　　B　✗　Usually 45, XO C ovarian dysgenesis
　　　C　✗　Secondary amenorrhoea or premature menopause usually
　　　D　✗　Impaired dihydrotestosterone production
　　　E　✔　Associated with reduced serum gonadotrophins and anosmia

7.13　A　✗　Werner's syndrome is inherited as an autosomal dominant trait
　　　B　✗　A recognized feature, e.g. acromegaly
　　　C　✔　Medullary thyroid carcinoma suggests MEN type II syndrome
　　　D　✗　Associated with gastrinomas (Zollinger–Ellison syndrome)
　　　E　✗　Associated with insulinomas

7.14　A　✗　Sipple's syndrome is also inherited as autosomal dominant
　　　B　✗　Associated with parathyroid adenoma, similar to MEN type I
　　　C　✗　Associated with medullary thyroid carcinoma
　　　D　✗　Multiple mucosal neurofibromata and marfanoid appearance
　　　E　✔　Not a recognized association with MEN syndromes

7.15 A ✔ Only adrenal phaeochromocytomas secrete adrenaline
      B ✘
      C ✘ Due to hypercalcaemia, parathyroid adenomas and MEN II
      D ✘ All 'typical' features of phaeochromocytoma
      E ✘ Catecholamines antagonize the actions of insulin

7.16 A ✔ The ratio is usually high
      B ✘ Gene defect increases intra-renal glucocorticoid levels
      C ✘
      D ✘ Dexamethasone reverses metabolic and hypertensive
             effects
      E ✘

7.17 A ✘ It is secreted by adipocytes and acts at a number of sites
             including the hypothalamus
      B ✘ It inhibits neuropeptide Y synthesis
      C ✔
      D ✘ Plasma levels are normal or high
      E ✘ It increases αMSH synthesis

7.18 A ✔ Raised plasma testosterone, oestrone and LH levels
      B ✘ LH:FSH ratio is typically >2.5
      C ✘ No change
      D ✘ But a mild increase in the plasma prolactin
      E ✘

7.19 A ✘ Raised in 2nd and 3rd trimesters
      B ✔
      C ✘
      D ✘ Typically rises throughout pregnancy
      E ✘ Raised

7.20 A ✘ Present in 10–30% of cases
      B ✔ Testes may be soft but are usually of normal size
      C ✘
      D ✘ Obesity is present in >70% of cases
      E ✘ Occurs in >80% of cases

7.21 A ✘ High serum alkaline phosphatase (ALP) levels
      B ✘ Low serum calcium and phosphate with high ALP
      C ✔ Inherited ALP deficiency — phosphates inhibit bone
             mineralization
      D ✘ High serum calcium and low serum phosphate levels
      E ✘ Usually high serum calcium but occasionally normal

7.22 A ✔ A complication of ulcerative colitis
      B ✘ May predate diabetes
      C ✘ Avoided by rotatation of insulin injection sites
      D ✘
      E ✘

7.23　A　✗
　　　B　✗
　　　C　✔　Unlike XXY; majority of patients have a normal phenotype
　　　D　✗　Especially in severe cardiac failure
　　　E　✗　XXY; occurs in hypergonadotrophic hypogonadism

7.24　A　✗　Urinary osmolality is high given a low plasma osmolality
　　　B　✗　Hyponatraemia stimulates aldosterone release; serum K is normal or low
　　　C　✗　Water is retained, not excreted
　　　D　✔　Small-cell lung carcinoma is the commonest cause
　　　E　✗　Plasma osmolality and blood urea are low

7.25　A　✔
　　　B　✗　An alkalosis is associated with hypokalaemia
　　　C　✗　Usually hyperkalaemia
　　　D　✗　An alkalosis due to acid losses in urine and vomit
　　　E　✗　Chronic respiratory acidosis

7.26　A　✗　Carbimazole blocks iodination of tyrosine
　　　B　✗　Not a contraindication; surgery may be more appropriate
　　　C　✗　Elevated free T_4 and low TSH
　　　D　✔　May predate thyrotoxicosis; in the elderly, eye signs are often absent
　　　E　✗　Propranolol reduces peripheral T_4 conversion to T_3

7.27　A　✗　Pallor is a striking feature of hypopituitarism
　　　B　✔　Amenorrhoea is a diagnostic feature of both conditions
　　　C　✗　Patients with anorexia nervosa have increased body hair (lanugo)
　　　D　✗　Adrenal function is normal in anorexia nervosa
　　　E　✗　Loss of body fat occurs in anorexia nervosa

7.28　A　✗　Especially if hypothermic
　　　B　✗
　　　C　✗　A visceral myopathy
　　　D　✗
　　　E　✔　The high plasma cholesterol reflects decreased utilization

7.29　A　✗　Due to tetany
　　　B　✗　Basal ganglia calcification
　　　C　✗
　　　D　✗　Occurs in 50% of cases
　　　E　✔　Common to the pseudohypoparathyroid syndromes

7.30 A ✗ Polyuria in diabetes is due to an osmotic diuresis; there will be glycosuria
B ✗ Hypercalcaemia causes nephrogenic diabetes insipidus
C ✗ Nephrogenic diabetes insipidus due to analgesic nephropathy
D ✗ Renal sarcoidosis or cerebral sarcoid would impair urinary concentration
E ✔

7.31 A ✗ The serum phosphate is low
B ✗ Urinary phosphate excretion is increased
C ✔ Thiazide diuretics may precipitate hypercalcaemia
D ✗ Prevalence 1:1000
E ✗ Asymptomatic individuals under 50 should have surgery

7.32 A ✗ Oligomenorrhoea is a more common finding
B ✗ Also hypothyroidism
C ✗ Hypopituitarism
D ✗
E ✔ Karyotype 45, XO gonadal dysgenesis

7.33 A ✗ Surgery is indicated if visual field defects are found
B ✔ Goitre is common in acromegaly
C ✗ Hypercalciuria in 50%
D ✗ Common and should be excluded especially with large tumours
E ✗ Usually due to an acidophil adenoma

7.34 A ✗ Most enzyme defects are autosomal recessive
B ✗ 17 hydroxyprogesterone is formed before enzyme block
C ✗ Typically absent
D ✔ Macrogenitosomia in the male infant is characteristic
E ✗ Clitoral hypertrophy and ambiguous genitalia in females

7.35 A ✔ TSH is suppressed and free T_4 elevated
B ✗ Medical and surgical therapy are equally effective
C ✗ Exophthalmos is more common in Graves' disease
D ✗ Typical of Graves' disease
E ✗

7.36 A ✗ Usually normal
B ✗ Increased
C ✗ 10- to 20-fold increase in females
D ✗ Usually suppressed
E ✔ But may be decreased

7.37 A ✗ 10% have diabetes
B ✗
C ✔
D ✗ MEN type II multiple endocrine neoplasia with a phaeochromocytoma
E ✗

7.38 A ✔ ADH secretion is inhibited by a rising blood alcohol level
     B ✘
     C ✘
     D ✘ Common postoperative phenomenon
     E ✘ Central effect; ADH is also stimulated by nausea

7.39 A ✘ Associated with increased iron deposits
     B ✔ Impaired glucose tolerance occurs in more than 80% of patients
     C ✘ A combination of testicular and pituitary impairment
     D ✘ Pseudogout is a typical feature
     E ✘ HLA A_3 positive in 70% of patients

7.40 A ✔ But seen in most other porphyrias
     B ✘ Contributing to acute neurological, psychiatric and GI disturbance
     C ✘
     D ✘ Increased delta-ALA synthetase activitity
     E ✘

8

Nephrology

QUESTIONS

8.1 Which ONE of the following statements about renal physiology in health is TRUE?
A Each kidney comprises approximately 5 million nephrons
B The kidneys receive approximately 5% of the cardiac output
C Variations in the calibre of afferent and efferent arterioles control the filtration pressure
D Anionic proteins are filtered more readily than cationic proteins
E Interstitial cells in the medulla are important in the production of erythropoietin

8.2 Which ONE of the following is most likely to be associated with oliguria?
A Poorly controlled diabetes mellitus
B Lithium therapy
C Chronic liver failure
D Addison's disease
E Hypercalcaemia

8.3 Which ONE of the following statements about urinary protein excretion is TRUE?
A Bence-Jones proteinuria is readily detectable using a dipstix testing
B Proteinuria >0.5 g/day is diagnostic of glomerulonephropathy
C Proteinuria is greater during the night than during the day
D Myoglobinuria is undetectable on dipstix testing for the presence of blood
E In early diabetic nephropathy, proteinuria predominantly comprises albumin

8.4 A 45-year-old man is found to have proteinuria in excess of 3.5 g per day at a 'routine' medical examination. Which ONE of the following diagnoses is the MOST likely?
A Cardiac failure
B Polycystic renal disease
C Renal amyloidosis
D Medullary cystic disease
E Chronic pyelonephritis

8.5   In a 40-year-old woman with microscopic haematuria, which ONE of the following disorders suggests that an alternative or additional diagnosis must be present to explain the urinary finding?
   A   Urinary tract infection
   B   Renal papillary necrosis
   C   Membranous glomerulonephritis
   D   Infective endocarditis
   E   Renal infarction

8.6   Which ONE of the following statements about the investigation of renal disease is TRUE?
   A   A random urinary pH of 4 suggests renal tubular acidosis
   B   Creatinine clearance reflects the ratio of the urinary and plasma concentrations
   C   Urinary albumin/creatinine ratio of 1 mg/mmol indicates glomerular disease
   D   A urinary protein/creatinine ratio of 50 (mg/mmol) indicates glomerular disease
   E   Renal biopsy should be undertaken in all patients with chronic renal failure

8.7   Which ONE of the following features would be an EXPECTED finding in a patient who has been diabetic for 15 years and who has more than 3 g proteinuria per day?
   A   Bilateral renal angle pain
   B   Unilateral left-sided pleural effusion
   C   Proteinuria 1.5 g/day
   D   Hypercholesterolaemia
   E   Urinary sodium concentration >20 mmol/L

8.8   In which ONE of the following disorders would renal biopsy be likely to show a focal segmental glomerulonephritis?
   A   Acute pyelonephritis
   B   Acute hepatitis A virus infection
   C   Microscopic polyarteritis nodosa
   D   Membranous nephropathy
   E   Renal amyloidosis

8.9   In an adolescent patient, which ONE of the following findings would be expected in acute, post-streptococcal glomerulonephritis?
   A   Hypotension
   B   Normal renal tubular function
   C   Hypercomplementaemia
   D   Polyuria
   E   Macroscopic haematuria

8.10 A young man presents with lethargy and is found to have moderate renal impairment. Which ONE of the following features suggests a mesangiocapillary nephropathy rather than an IgA nephropathy?
A   Recurrent macroscopic haematuria
B   Onset 3–7 days after a respiratory tract infection
C   An association with Henoch–Schönlein purpura
D   An association with partial lipodystrophy
E   Mesangial cell proliferation on renal biopsy

8.11 Which ONE of the following features suggests Goodpasture's disease?
A   Circulating anti-neutrophil cytoplasmic antibodies (c-ANCA or anti-PR3)
B   Mesangial IgA deposition
C   Presentation with the nephrotic syndrome
D   Haemoptysis and pulmonary infiltrates on chest X-ray
E   Association with HLA-DR3

8.12 Which ONE of the following features is characteristic of minimal change nephropathy?
A   Occurrence in adults usually follows an acute infection
B   Marked mesangial cell proliferation on renal biopsy
C   Nephrotic syndrome with unselective proteinuria
D   Hypertension and microscopic haematuria
E   The absence of impaired renal function

8.13 Which ONE of the following statements about the treatment of minimal change nephropathy is TRUE?
A   Therapy should be deferred pending renal biopsy in childhood
B   Diuretics should be avoided to minimize the risk of renal impairment
C   Following remission, more than one third of patients relapse within 3 years
D   Immunosuppressant therapy is unlikely to prevent further relapses
E   Impaired renal function eventually develops if relapses are frequent

8.14 Which ONE of the following features is characteristic of renal tubular acidosis (RTA)?
A   An anion gap >15 mmol/L
B   Hyperchloraemic acidosis
C   Urinary pH <5.4
D   Decreased glomerular filtration rate
E   Normocytic normochromic anaemia

8.15 Which ONE of the following features is characteristic of an acute interstitial nephritis?
A   Skin rashes, arthralgia and fever
B   Peripheral blood eosinophilia
C   Renal biopsy evidence of an eosinophilic interstitial nephritis
D   Renal impairment typically follows withdrawal of the drug
E   Onset following an acute emotional distress

8.16 Which ONE of the following findings indicates a diagnosis of pre-renal rather than established acute renal failure?
A   Oliguria <700 ml per day
B   Urine/plasma urea ratio <10:1
C   A urinary osmolality >600 mosmol/kg
D   A urinary sodium concentration >20 mmol/L
E   Hypertension rather than hypotension

8.17 In a previously healthy adolescent girl, which ONE of the following features is most consistent with a diagnosis of a lower urinary tract infection?
A   Rigors, loin pain and renal impairment
B   Suprapubic pain, dysuria and haematuria
C   Progression to acute pyelonephritis if untreated
D   Midstream urine culture producing *Escherichia coli* 10 000/ml
E   Ciprofloxacin is the drug of choice in the majority of patients

8.18 Which ONE of the following statements about urinary tract infection during pregnancy is TRUE?
A   Asymptomatic bacteriuria is present in 50% of patients
B   Ureteric atonia predisposes to the onset of acute pyelonephritis
C   Treatment of asymptomatic bacteriuria is contraindicated until symptoms occur
D   Intravenous urography is mandatory if acute pyelonephritis ensues
E   Trimethoprim is the treatment of choice in acute cystitis

8.19 A 45-year-old woman presents with tiredness with a plasma creatinine of 450 μmol/L. Which ONE of the following findings would be EXPECTED in chronic renal failure?
A   Normal urinary concentrating ability
B   Hypophosphataemia
C   Hypercalcaemia
D   Metabolic acidosis
E   Proteinuria >3.5 g/day

8.20 A 45-year-old man presents with severe right-sided loin pain. A plain abdominal X-ray suggests a calculus in the region of the right kidney. Which ONE of the following statements about the treatment of renal calculi is TRUE?
- **A** Anuria indicates the need for urgent surgical intervention
- **B** The urine should be alkalinized if the stone is radio-opaque
- **C** Bendroflumethiazide (bendrofluazide) usefully increases urinary calcium excretion
- **D** Allopurinol increases urinary urate excretion in patients with chronic gout
- **E** Renal pelvic stones are best removed by open surgery

8.21 Which ONE of the following features suggests an alternative diagnosis to that of adult polycystic renal disease?
- **A** Sex-linked recessive mode of inheritance
- **B** Cystic disease of the liver and pancreas
- **C** Renal angle pain and haematuria
- **D** Aortic and mitral regurgitation
- **E** Aneurysms of the circle of Willis

8.22 Which ONE of the following features is a typical finding in bladder carcinoma?
- **A** Squamous cell rather than transitional cell in origin
- **B** Presentation with urinary frequency and nocturia
- **C** Unresponsive to radiotherapy
- **D** Early metastatic spread to the liver and lungs
- **E** Association with exposure to dyes and tobacco consumption

8.23 Which ONE of the following features would be a typical feature at presentation in a patient with benign prostatic hypertrophy (BPH)?
- **A** Peak incidence in the age group 40–60 years
- **B** Microscopic haematuria
- **C** Increased plasma testosterone concentration
- **D** Normal serum prostatic acid phosphatase concentration
- **E** Asymmetrical prostatic enlargement on rectal examination

8.24 Which ONE of the following features is typical in a patient with prostatic carcinoma?
- **A** Rapidly progressive chronic renal failure
- **B** Slowly progressive urinary frequency
- **C** Preservation of the normal anatomy on digital rectal examination
- **D** Distal rather than local dissemination of the tumour
- **E** Osteolytic rather than osteosclerotic bone metastases

8.25 Which ONE of the following statements about testicular tumours is TRUE?
- **A** Seminoma of the testis usually presents with testicular pain
- **B** Teratomas secrete alpha-foetoprotein and chorionic gonadotrophin
- **C** Metastatic spread occurs exclusively via the lymphatic system
- **D** The peak incidence occurs after the age of 60 years
- **E** Seminomas are radio-resistant but chemo-sensitive

ANSWERS

8.1   A   ✘   One million nephrons per kidney
     B   ✘   25% of the cardiac output
     C   ✔
     D   ✘   Cationic proteins are more readily filtered
     E   ✘   They produce prostaglandins; cortical fibroblasts produce erythropoietin

8.2   A   ✘   Hyperglycaemia causes an osmotic diuresis
     B   ✘   Causes nephrogenic diabetes insipidus
     C   ✔   Excess antidiuretic hormone (ADH) and the hepato-renal syndrome
     D   ✘   Mineralocorticoid deficiency impairs urinary concentrating ability
     E   ✘   Causes nephrogenic diabetes insipidus

8.3   A   ✘   Immunoelectrophoresis required
     B   ✘   >3.5 g/day often with oedema and hypoalbuminaemia
     C   ✘   Greater when upright — 'orthostatic proteinuria'
     D   ✘   Labstix test positive but no red cells on microscopy
     E   ✔   Microalbuminuria is a sensitive predictor

8.4   A   ✘   Moderate 500 mg–2 g — rarely more
     B   ✘   Usually haematuria
     C   ✔
     D   ✘   Causes polyuria and renal failure
     E   ✘   No glomerular lesion

8.5   A   ✘
     B   ✘   Factors include diabetes mellitus, chronic NSAID abuse and alcoholism
     C   ✔   Typically proteinuria alone
     D   ✘   Associated with a mesangiocapillary glomerulonephritis
     E   ✘   May also cause macroscopic haematuria

8.6   A   ✘   RTA produces an inability to acidify urine (pH >8 suggests infection)
     B   ✔   C = urine concentration/plasma concentration × urine volume
     C   ✘   Glomerular disease is likely if the ratio >3.5 mg/mmol
     D   ✘   Glomerular disease is likely if the ratio >300
     E   ✘   Contraindicated if both kidneys are small (<60% normal size)

8.7   A   ✘   Typically painless
     B   ✘   Usually right-sided or bilateral effusions
     C   ✘   Serum albumin concentration <30 g/L and urinary protein >3.0 g/day
     D   ✔   Producing progressive atherosclerosis
     E   ✘   Marked sodium retention — urinary sodium <10 mmol/L

8.8   A   ✗   Tubulointerstitial damage only
      B   ✗   Acute hepatitis B virus infection; also a feature of HIV
              infection
      C   ✔   Typical of small vessel vasculitis
      D   ✗   Presents with nephritic syndrome
      E   ✗   Characterized by immunoglobulin light chain deposition

8.9   A   ✗   Hypertension
      B   ✔
      C   ✗   'Classical' pathway activation producing
              hypocomplementaemia
      D   ✗   Oedema and oliguria are typical
      E   ✗   Microscopic haematuria with red cell casts on microscopy

8.10 A   ✗   Suggests IgA nephropathy
      B   ✗   Suggests IgA nephropathy
      C   ✗   Suggests IgA nephropathy
      D   ✔   And chronic Hepatitis B viral infection
      E   ✗   Suggests IgA nephropathy

8.11 A   ✗   Circulating anti-glomerular basement membrane
              antibodies
      B   ✗   Crescentic nephritis with linear IgG deposition
      C   ✗   Presentation with acute renal failure
      D   ✔   Antibodies have pulmonary basement membrane cross-
              reactivity
      E   ✗   HLA-DR15; HLA-DR3 is associated with membranous
              glomerulopathy

8.12 A   ✗   Usually children; accounts for 25% of nephrotic syndrome
              in adults
      B   ✗   Minor or absent
      C   ✗   Selective proteinuria
      D   ✗   Suggests an alternative cause
      E   ✔   Renal function is unimpaired

8.13 A   ✗   Diagnosis in children rarely requires histological
              confirmation
      B   ✗   Useful in management of oedema
      C   ✔   Longer term steroids may be helpful
      D   ✗   Cyclophosphamide can help prevent frequent relapses
      E   ✗   Rarely, even in relapsing disease

8.14 A   ✗   Normal anion gap $(Na^+ + K^+) - (Cl^- + HCO3^-)$; normally <15
              mmol/L
      B   ✔   Increased chloride preserves anion gap
      C   ✗   Urinary pH is inappropriately >5.4 even in presence of
              systemic acidosis
      D   ✗   GFR is normal
      E   ✗   No features of uraemia

8.15 A ✘ Less than 30% of drug-induced AIN have generalized hypersensitivity
 B ✘ Eosinophilia occurs in 30% in the peripheral blood and 70% in the urine
 C ✔ And neutrophil or monocytic infiltrate
 D ✘ Typically resolves
 E ✘ Onset after exposure to drug therapy, especially penicillin or NSAIDs

8.16 A ✘ 20% of acute renal failure is non-oliguric
 B ✘ U/P ratio >10:1 indicating good renal medullary function
 C ✔ Indicating preservation of renal medullary function
 D ✘ Urinary sodium <20 mmol/L indicates normal renal medullary function
 E ✘ Suggests primary renal disease

8.17 A ✘ Suggests acute pyelonephritis
 B ✔ And urinary frequency
 C ✘ Suggests an abnormality of the urinary tract
 D ✘ *E. coli* >100 000/ml suggests infection (75% of UTIs in the community)
 E ✘ Trimethoprim or co-amoxiclav pending the results of bacterial sensitivities

8.18 A ✘ 5% cf. 40% in elderly females
 B ✔ And ureteric dilatation
 C ✘ 40% of patients with untreated asymptomatic bacteriuria will develop UTI
 D ✘ Contraindicated in early pregnancy
 E ✘ Teratogenic risk (a folate antagonist)

8.19 A ✘ Polyuria due to impaired renal medullary function
 B ✘ Hyperphosphataemia
 C ✘ Hypocalcaemia
 D ✔ Resulting in hyperpnoea
 E ✘ Severe proteinuria diminishes as renal failure progresses

8.20 A ✔ Suggests total obstruction
 B ✘ Acidification with ammonium chloride may benefit
 C ✘ Decreases urinary calcium excretion by 30% in hypercalciuric patients
 D ✘ Decreases urinary urate and may reduce oxalate stone formation
 E ✘ Fragmentation by lithotripsy and endoscopic removal is possible

8.21 A ✔ Autosomal dominant inheritance
 B ✘ But liver function tests normal
 C ✘ Hypertension and UTI are also common at presentation
 D ✘ Common but rarely severe
 E ✘ 10% will have a subarachnoid haemorrhage

8.22　A　✗　Typically transitional cell
　　　B　✗　Painless haematuria is typical
　　　C　✗　Radiotherapy is of palliative benefit
　　　D　✗　Local spread occurs early and metastases late
　　　E　✔　Also associated with chronic schistosomiasis

8.23　A　✗　Aged over 60 years
　　　B　✗　Urinary frequency and nocturia sometimes precipitated by UTI
　　　C　✗　Associated with diminished androgen secretion
　　　D　✔　Even modest changes may herald prostatic carcinoma
　　　E　✗　Typically symmetrical

8.24　A　✗　Slowly progressive obstructive uropathy similar to BPH
　　　B　✔　And nocturia or haematuria
　　　C　✗　Hard with obliteration of median furrow
　　　D　✗　Usually local spread then distal spread to bones
　　　E　✗　Osteosclerotic metastases

8.25　A　✗　Typically a painless swelling of the testis
　　　B　✔　Helps in the assessment of treatment response
　　　C　✗　Haematogenous spread may occur
　　　D　✗　Peak incidence aged 25–34 years
　　　E　✗　Sensitive to both radiotherapy and chemotherapy

9

Neurology

QUESTIONS

9.1 **Which ONE of the following statements about neurophysiological investigations is TRUE?**
A The dominant rhythm on the EEG in health is the theta rhythm
B The alpha rhythm persists when the eyes are closed
C The EEG is usually abnormal between seizures
D The normal conduction velocity in motor nerves is 5–6 m/s
E Metabolic myopathies are characterized by normal EMG findings

9.2 **Which ONE of the following statements about neuroradiological investigations is TRUE?**
A CT scanning is preferred for visualization of the posterior fossa
B MR imaging provides more detailed analysis of grey but not white matter
C CT scanning is preferred in the examination of the orbit
D MR imaging avoids exposure to ionizing radiation
E Inter-observer variability is low in carotid Doppler ultrasound

9.3 **A 17-year-old presents with an acute headache and undergoes lumbar puncture. Which ONE of the following is a 'normal' finding on cerebrospinal fluid analysis?**
A An opening pressure = 190 mm/H_2O
B A glucose content <25% of the plasma concentration
C A protein content 0.8 g/L
D A white cell count 10 cells/mm^3
E Absence of oligoclonal IgG bands

9.4 **In which ONE of the following disorders would the finding of dysphonia suggest an alternative diagnosis?**
A Myasthenia gravis
B Supranuclear bulbar palsy
C Parkinson's disease
D Cerebellar disease
E Lesion of Broca's area

9.5   In which ONE of the following disorders would the finding of
dysarthria suggest an alternative diagnosis?
A   Bilateral recurrent laryngeal nerve palsies
B   Supranuclear bulbar palsy
C   Cerebellar disease
D   Myasthenia gravis
E   Bulbar palsy

9.6   Which ONE of the following findings suggests an alternative or
additional diagnosis to that of an upper motor neurone disorder?
A   Extensor plantar responses
B   Absent abdominal reflexes
C   Muscle fasciculation
D   Increased tendon reflexes
E   Plantar flexion of the great toe in response to rapid
dorsiflexion of the toes

9.7   Which ONE of the following findings suggests an alternative or
additional diagnosis to that of a lower motor neurone disorder?
A   Flaccid muscle tone
B   The rapid onset of muscle wasting
C   Absent or decreased tendon reflexes
D   Muscle fasciculation
E   Extensor plantar responses

9.8   Which ONE of the following findings suggests an alternative or
additional diagnosis to that of extrapyramidal tract disease?
A   'Clasp-knife' rigidity
B   Delayed initiation of movements
C   Choreo-athetosis
D   Delayed relaxation of the tendon reflexes
E   Coarse tremor at a rate of 3 cycles per second

9.9   Which ONE of the following statements about the lateral
spinothalamic tract of the spinal cord is TRUE?
A   It transmits pain sensation from the same side of the body
B   It crosses to the opposite side in the medial lemniscus
C   It transmits contralateral light touch sensation
D   It stratifies fibres from the lowest spinal segments innermost
E   It crosses from the thalamus to the contralateral parietal lobe

9.10   In which ONE of the following disorders is the loss of tendon
reflexes a predominant clinical finding?
A   Proximal myopathy
B   Transverse myelitis
C   Syringomyelia
D   Myasthenia gravis
E   Motor neurone disease

9.11 **Which ONE of the following statements about bladder innervation is TRUE?**
  A   Sacral cord lesions usually produce urinary retention
  B   Thoracic cord lesions are not typically associated with urinary problems
  C   Sympathetic stimulation causes bladder emptying
  D   Pudendal nerve lesions typically produce automatic bladder emptying
  E   The sympathetic outflow to the bladder arises from the S1–S2 segment

9.12 **Which ONE of the following findings suggests an alternative or additional diagnosis to that of cerebellar disease?**
  A   Dysmetria
  B   Dysarthria
  C   Intention tremor
  D   Decreased muscle tone
  E   Pendular nystagmus

9.13 **A 75-year-old man presents having noticed impaired sensation of the left side of his face while shaving. Which ONE of the following diagnoses can be excluded as the cause of his complaint?**
  A   Cavernous sinus disease
  B   Trigeminal neuralgia
  C   Acoustic neuroma
  D   Lesion of the posterior limb of the right internal capsule
  E   Lesion of the upper cervical cord segments

9.14 **A 45-year-old obese woman presents with a history of blurred vision and is found to have bilateral papilloedema on ophthalmoscopy. Which ONE of the following diagnoses can be excluded as the cause of her complaint?**
  A   Migraine
  B   Cavernous sinus thrombosis
  C   Hypertension
  D   Chronic ventilatory failure
  E   Cerebral abscess

9.15 **In which ONE of the following disorders would the finding of muscle fasciculation of the tongue suggest an alternative or additional diagnosis to the diagnoses listed below?**
  A   Pseudobulbar palsy
  B   Syringobulbia
  C   Motor neurone disease
  D   Nasopharyngeal carcinoma
  E   Paget's disease of the skull

9.16 In a patient with temporal lobe epilepsy, which ONE of the following findings would suggest an additional diagnosis?
A Complex partial seizure with loss of awareness
B Hallucinations of smell, taste, hearing or vision
C *Déjà vu* phenomena associated with intense emotion
D Progression to tonic-clonic seizure
E EEG shows spike and wave activity at 3 cycles/second

9.17 Which ONE of the following statements about the management of tonic-clonic epilepsy is TRUE?
A All patients should be admitted to hospital following a first seizure
B Patients may safely return to car driving after 1 year free from seizures
C A heavy goods vehicle driving licence will be revoked until 3 years free from seizures
D Anticonvulsant therapy should be started after the first proven seizure
E The use of two or more anticonvulsant drugs is preferable to monotherapy

9.18 Which ONE of the following findings suggests that the finding of papilloedema is likely to be due to raised intracranial pressure?
A Severe visual impairment at presentation
B An arcuate scotoma progressing to 'tunnel' vision
C Pain and tenderness in the affected eye
D Retinal haemorrhages close to the optic disc if rapid in onset
E Ipsilateral optic atrophy in tumours of the anterior cranial fossa

9.19 In a patient presenting with recurrent headaches, which ONE of the following features MOST suggests the diagnosis of migraine?
A Absence of a family history of migraine
B Onset before the age of puberty
C Headache is unilateral and always on the same side of the head
D Premonitory symptoms include teichopsia
E Hemiparaesthesiae persisting for several weeks after the attack

9.20 In which ONE of the following disorders would the risk of anticoagulation be significantly greater than the risk of cerebral embolism from the underlying disorder?
A Mechanical prosthetic mitral valve
B Atrial fibrillation associated with rheumatic mitral valve disease
C Left atrial myxoma
D Infective endocarditis of the aortic valve
E Myocardial infarction with left ventricular mural thrombus

9.21 In a patient presenting with a diagnosis of brain stem infarction, which ONE of the following features would suggest an additional or alternative diagnosis?
   A   Pin-point pupils
   B   Vertigo and diplopia
   C   Sensory dysphasia
   D   Severe headache
   E   Bidirectional jerking nystagmus

9.22 A 72-year-old right-handed lady is admitted with collapse and new onset upper motor neurone weakness. Which ONE of the following features suggests a good prognosis?
   A   Coma persisting for more than 24 hours
   B   Haemorrhagic stroke rather than an embolic stoke
   C   Absence of hypertension immediately following the stroke
   D   Presence of a conjugate gaze palsy
   E   Left-sided rather than right-sided hemiplegia

9.23 Which ONE of the following features is the most typical finding in chronic subdural haematoma?
   A   Recall of a recent head injury
   B   Urinary incontinence and ataxia
   C   Epilepsy without previous headaches
   D   Hemiplegia and hemianopia of sudden onset
   E   Absence of impaired consciousness

9.24 Which ONE of the following features is the most typical finding in herpes zoster?
   A   A rash that heals without scarring
   B   Permanent dermatomal sensory impairment
   C   Infection is confined to the posterior root ganglia
   D   A rash appears 1–2 days before the onset of pain
   E   Treatment with aciclovir prevents post-herpetic neuralgia

9.25 In a 29-year-old homosexual patient with known syphilis, which ONE of the following findings suggests the presence of an additional, unrelated diagnosis?
   A   Septic meningitis
   B   Pre-senile dementia
   C   Hemiplegia
   D   Truncal ataxia
   E   Trigeminal neuralgia

9.26 In a patient suspected of having tabes dorsalis, which ONE of the following findings suggests an alternative diagnosis?
   A   Paroxysmal abdominal and girdle pains
   B   Loss of pain sensation of the nose, perineum and lower limbs
   C   Bilateral ptosis and absent pupillary light reflexes
   D   Increased knee and ankle reflexes with extensor plantar responses
   E   High-stepping gait with muscle hypotonia

9.27 Which ONE of the following statements about multiple sclerosis is TRUE?

A   It predominantly affects young males
B   It is associated with HLA B27 haplotype
C   It has a prevalence of about 80 per 100 000 of the UK population
D   It is more prevalent in the tropics than in temperate climates
E   Demyelinating plaques within the CNS are confined to the grey matter

9.28 In a patient presenting with parkinsonian features, which ONE of the following factors can be excluded as an aetological factor?

A   Progressive supranuclear palsy
B   Long-term phenothiazine therapy
C   Haemochromatosis
D   Repetitive head injury in boxers
E   Methyl-phenyl-tetrahydropyridine exposure

9.29 Which ONE of the following clinical findings is MOST consistent with a diagnosis of idiopathic Parkinson's disease?

A   Unilateral onset of the disorder
B   Emotional lability
C   Oculogyric crises
D   Extensor plantar responses
E   Impaired voluntary eye movements

9.30 Which ONE of the following statements about the management of Parkinson's disease is TRUE?

A   Anticholinergic therapy is the best first line therapy for hypokinesis
B   L-dopa should be introduced as soon as diagnosis is made
C   Sialorrhoea invariably indicates overuse of L-dopa
D   Dopamine receptor agonists, unlike anticholinergics, do not cause confusion
E   Dyskinesia is a frequent dose-limiting side effect of L-dopa

9.31 Which ONE of the following findings is MOST consistent with hemisection of the spinal cord (Brown-Séquard syndrome)?

A   Pain and temperature sensory loss in the ipsilateral leg
B   Proprioceptive sensory loss in the contralateral leg
C   An extensor plantar response in the ipsilateral leg
D   Hyperreflexia and weakness of the contralateral leg
E   Hyperaesthetic dermatome on the opposite side of the lesion

9.32 Which ONE of the following statements about the treatment of established paraplegia is TRUE?
A Prophylactic antibiotics are of no proven value in the prevention of recurrent urinary sepsis
B Pressure sores are not likely to occur unless sensation is lost
C Urinary retention usually requires long-term catheterization
D Flexor spasms and contractures are usually unavoidable
E Constipation requires dietary treatment and regular enemas

9.33 In a patient presenting with neurological dysfunction, the serum vitamin B_{12} level is found to be significantly decreased. Which ONE of the following features on clinical examination suggests that the vitamin B_{12} deficiency may be unrelated to the neurological disorder?
A Mononeuritis multiplex
B Optic atrophy
C Confusion and dementia
D Spastic paraparesis
E Sensory ataxia

9.34 Which ONE of the following features is most consistent with the diagnosis of carpal tunnel syndrome?
A Remission during pregnancy
B Wasting of the dorsal interossei and lumbricals
C Pain in the hand which is worse by day rather than by night
D Association with hyperthyroidism
E Complication of both rheumatoid arthritis and amyloidosis

9.35 Which ONE of the following patterns of sensory loss correctly identifies a lesion of the peripheral nerves listed below?
A Lateral palm and thumb, index and half of ring finger — ulnar nerve
B Medial palm and little finger, half ring finger — median nerve
C Palmar aspect of the thumb — radial nerve
D Dorsum of foot — lateral interosseous nerve
E Lateral border of thigh — obturator nerve

9.36 In a patient suspected as having the Duchenne type of muscular dystrophy, which ONE of the following features suggests an alternative diagnosis?
A Symptoms and signs presenting in the third year of life
B Evidence of calf muscle hypertrophy
C Difficulty in rising from the floor
D Normal serum creatine phosphokinase concentration
E Development of respiratory failure during late adolescence

9.37 **In a patient suspected as having myasthenia gravis, which ONE of the following features suggests an alternative diagnosis?**
A Absent knee jerks that reappear immediately after sustained quadriceps contraction
B Circulating anti-acetylcholine receptor antibodies
C Onset of the disease between the ages of 15 and 50 years
D Absence of muscle wasting
E Intermittent diplopia and ptosis

9.38 **Which ONE of the following statements about the treatment of myasthenia gravis is TRUE?**
A Pupillary miosis, salivation and sweating suggest insufficient drug therapy
B Pyridostigmine therapy is best given with propantheline once per day
C Thymectomy should be deferred for as long as possible after the onset of therapy
D Corticosteroid therapy produces a transient myasthenic crisis
E The prognosis is significantly better if associated with a thymoma

9.39 **Which ONE of the following statements about the Glasgow coma scale is TRUE?**
A The average response to an arousal stimulus should be measured
B Appropriate motor responses to verbal commands = score 4
C Spontaneous eye opening = score 4
D Verbal responses with normal speech and orientation = score 6
E The minimum total score = 6

9.40 **Which ONE of the following features supports the diagnosis of brain stem death?**
A Pin-point pupils
B Persistent corneal reflexes
C Absence of eye movement responses to ice cold water in either ear
D Development of periodic respiration
E Preservation of the cough and gag reflexes

ANSWERS

9.1   A   ✗   The alpha rhythm; lower frequencies predominate during sleep
      B   ✗   It disappears
      C   ✗   Normal in 50%
      D   ✗   50–60 m/s
      E   ✔   There is no change in muscle fibre structure

9.2   A   ✗   MRI provides more detail
      B   ✗   Better for both
      C   ✗   MRI provides more detail
      D   ✔   In contrast to CT
      E   ✗   Highly operator dependent

9.3   A   ✗   Opening pressure >180 mm/H_2O indicates raised intracranial pressure
      B   ✗   >60% of blood level
      C   ✗   The protein content is usually <0.5 g/L
      D   ✗   The normal white cell count is usually <4 mm^3
      E   ✔   Oligoclonal IgG bands suggest multiple sclerosis

9.4   A   ✗   Typically intermittent
      B   ✗   With dysarthria and dysphagia
      C   ✗   Soft, rapid, indistinct speech
      D   ✗   Scanning dysarthria
      E   ✔   Expressive dysphasia

9.5   A   ✔   Dysphonia
      B   ✗   Often due to cerebrovascular disease
      C   ✗   'Scanning' dysarthria
      D   ✗   In addition to dysphonia
      E   ✗

9.6   A   ✗   Flexor or absent in lower motor neurone lesion
      B   ✗   Segmental level T8–T12
      C   ✔   Lower motor neurone sign
      D   ✗   'Clasp-knife' rigidity is typical
      E   ✗   Rossolimo's sign

9.7   A   ✗   Increased in upper motor neurone lesions
      B   ✗
      C   ✗   With flexor or absent plantar response
      D   ✗
      E   ✔   Upper motor neurone lesion

9.8   A   ✔   'Lead pipe' or 'cog-wheel' rigidity
      B   ✗   Also other involuntary movements
      C   ✗   Hypothyroidism
      D   ✗   Hypokinesis
      E   ✗   Resting tremor

9.9   A   ✗   Opposite side
       B   ✗   Decussate below this level
       C   ✔   And temperature sensation
       D   ✗   Lowest segments outermost
       E   ✗   No decussation at this level

9.10   A   ✗   Reflexes preserved
       B   ✗   Reflexes enhanced below the level of the lesion
       C   ✔   At least one of the upper limb reflexes is lost
       D   ✗   Reflexes preserved
       E   ✗   Reflexes are increased

9.11   A   ✔   Due to parasympathetic denervation
       B   ✗   Produce urinary urge incontinence and incomplete bladder emptying
       C   ✗   Parasympathetic mediates internal sphincter relaxation and detrusor contraction
       D   ✗   Feature of spinal cord lesions
       E   ✗   Sympathetic outflow arises from the L1–L2 segment

9.12   A   ✗   'Past pointing'
       B   ✗   With loss of normal rhythm
       C   ✗   Absent at rest
       D   ✗   Hypotonia
       E   ✔   If present, nystagmus is normally jerking, not pendular

9.13   A   ✗   Ophthalmic and maxillary divisions of fifth nerve
       B   ✔   Facial pain without sensory loss
       C   ✗   In cerebellopontine angle
       D   ✗   Contralateral to site of loss
       E   ✗   Unilateral or bilateral

9.14   A   ✔   Suggests more sinister cause for headache
       B   ✗
       C   ✗   Grade 4 retinopathy
       D   ✗   With hypercapnia
       E   ✗   Raised intracranial pressure

9.15   A   ✔   Bilateral supranuclear lesions cause a spastic tongue
       B   ✗   Causing dysarthria, dysphonia and dysphagia
       C   ✗   Without any sensory involvement from bulbar palsy
       D   ✗   Invasion of the base of the skull
       E   ✗   Causes stenosis of hypoglossal canal

9.16   A   ✗   With automatic movements (e.g. lip-smacking)
       B   ✗   May be detailed with graphic descriptions
       C   ✗   Or *jamais vu* (unreality)
       D   ✗   In the minority
       E   ✔   Typical of petit mal epilepsy

9.17 A ✘ Admit if in status epilepticus or if there is a rapid recurrence
B ✔ Or 3 years of nocturnal seizures only
C ✘ Not until 10 years free of seizures whilst on NO anticonvulsant therapy
D ✘ Depends on the risk of recurrence and the presence of underlying disease
E ✘ Monotherapy is preferable

9.18 A ✘ Suggests optic neuritis
B ✘ Suggests chronic glaucoma
C ✘ Suggests optic neuritis
D ✔ Causes visual impairment
E ✘ Contralateral optic atrophy (Foster Kennedy syndrome)

9.19 A ✘ Positive family history in more than 50% of sufferers
B ✘ Typically post-pubertal
C ✘ Headache may become generalized and is rarely fixed to one side
D ✔ Visual scintillations and also fortification spectra and scotomas
E ✘ Focal deficits may occasionally persist 1–2 days but rarely longer

9.20 A ✘
B ✘ 33% incidence of embolism over 10 years untreated
C ✘
D ✔ Major risk of mycotic aneurysms and cerebral abscesses
E ✘ Occasionally if there is atrial fibrillation

9.21 A ✘ Especially pontine lesions
B ✘ With demonstrable third, fourth or sixth nerve lesions
C ✔ A cortical sign
D ✘ Often with vomiting
E ✘ Central type of jerking nystagmus

9.22 A ✘ Worse if the coma is prolonged
B ✘ Early mortality is higher in haemorrhagic stroke
C ✔ Hypertension suggests raised intracranial pressure or brain stem involvement
D ✘ Poor prognosis if persistent
E ✘ Functional outcome is worse with strokes of the non-dominant hemisphere

9.23 A ✘ Most have no history of trauma
B ✔ Slowly progressive
C ✘ Late-onset epilepsy suggests intracerebral disease
D ✘ Suggests cerebral infarction or haemorrhage
E ✘ Fluctuating confusional state and impairment of consciousness

9.24 A ✗ Marked post inflammatory depigmentation may occur
     B ✔ Sometimes with dysaesthesia
     C ✗ Rarely anterior (motor) ganglia involved
     D ✗ Rash follows onset of pain in 3–4 days; initial diagnosis may be difficult
     E ✗ May limit severity and duration of initial illness

9.25 A ✗ Secondary syphilis
     B ✗ Remember HIV infection
     C ✗ Secondary syphilis
     D ✗ Tabes dorsalis
     E ✔

9.26 A ✗ 'Lightning pains'
     B ✗ With trophic ulceration and Charcot joints
     C ✗ Argyll Robertson pupils and optic atrophy
     D ✔ But plantar responses may be extensor with taboparesis
     E ✗ Typical in sensory ataxia

9.27 A ✗ More women than men are affected
     B ✗ Association with HLA-A3, B7 and Dw2/DR2 in the UK
     C ✔ Highest prevalence is in the north-east of Scotland
     D ✗ The prevalence varies with latitude, being lowest in equatorial areas
     E ✗ Central white matter

9.28 A ✗ Conjugate gaze palsy affecting vertical eye movements
     B ✗ Other involuntary movement disorders
     C ✔ Unlike Wilson's disease
     D ✗ 'Punch drunk' syndrome
     E ✗ Used in herbicides and associated with extra-pyramidal disorders

9.29 A ✔ Typically arm tremor
     B ✗ Suggests underlying cerebrovascular disease
     C ✗ Suggests drug-induced extrapyramidal disease
     D ✗ Suggests multisystems atrophy (MSA)
     E ✗ Impairment of conjugate eye movements suggests progressive supranuclear palsy

9.30 A ✗ Principally useful for tremor
     B ✗ Early introduction means earlier waning of effect
     C ✗ May be a sign of undertreatment also
     D ✗ Neuropsychiatric problems occur with both types of therapy
     E ✔ Sustained-release preparations sometimes help

9.31 A ✗ Contralateral leg — spinothalamic tracts decussate after entering the spinal cord
    B ✗ Ipsilateral leg with dorsal column involvement
    C ✔ Pyramidal tract involvement
    D ✗ No contralateral pyramidal signs
    E ✗ Ipsilateral dermatomal sensory changes

9.32 A ✗ Guided by sensitivities of colonizing organisms
    B ✗ Immobility in itself predisposes to sore formation
    C ✗ Intermittent catheterization is usually preferrable
    D ✗ Good posturing and passive movement can minimize risk
    E ✔ Manual evacuation may be necessary

9.33 A ✔ Causes peripheral neuropathy
    B ✗ Typically bilateral and associated with abnormal cyanide metabolism
    C ✗ Often reversible
    D ✗ Pyramidal tract degeneration
    E ✗ Proprioceptive loss due to dorsal column disease (SACD)

9.34 A ✗ Often develops or worsens with pregnancy
    B ✗ Supplied by the ulnar nerve
    C ✗ Radiates up the arm and even to the shoulder
    D ✗ Associated with acromegaly and hypothyroidism
    E ✔ And previous wrist fracture

9.35 A ✗ Median nerve
    B ✗ Ulnar nerve
    C ✗ Dorsum of the thumb, often with weakness of wrist extension
    D ✔ The common peroneal nerve — often with a foot drop
    E ✗ Lateral cutaneous nerve of thigh

9.36 A ✗ As late as 10 years of age
    B ✗ With preserved tendon reflexes
    C ✗ Characteristic finding — Gowers' sign
    D ✔ Serum CK is raised from birth
    E ✗ Often associated with cardiac disease

9.37 A ✔ Characteristic of the Lambert–Eaton syndrome
    B ✗ 80% have ACh receptor antibodies
    C ✗ Especially occurs in females more than males
    D ✗ Wasting only occurs in severe, chronic disease
    E ✗ Often more marked in the evenings or following exercise

9.38 A ✗ 'Cholinergic crisis' due to excessive drug therapy
    B ✗ Best given every 3–6 hours
    C ✗ Best undertaken as soon as possible after the diagnosis is confirmed
    D ✔ Initiation of therapy is best undertaken in hospital
    E ✗ Worse, even after the thymoma is removed

9.39 A ✘ Test at least twice and measure the BEST response
      B ✘ No response to pain = 1; maximum score = 6
      C ✔ No eye opening = 1
      D ✘ No speech = 1; maximum score = 5
      E ✘ Minimum score = 3; maximum score = 15

9.40 A ✘ Pupils are fixed and dilated (unreactive to light)
      B ✘ Brain stem reflex is lost
      C ✔ Vestibulo-ocular responses to caloric testing are brain stem reflexes
      D ✘ Absence of spontaneous respiration ($PaCO_2$ >6.7 KPa)
      E ✘ All brain stem reflexes absent

10

Respiratory medicine

QUESTIONS

10.1 A 45-year-old woman presents with a 6-month history of breathlessness. Pulmonary function tests show an INCREASED transfer factor for carbon monoxide (TCO). Which ONE of the following disorders is the most likely explanation?
A Emphysema
B Thyrotoxicosis
C Fibrosing alveolitis
D Anaemia
E Chronic bronchitis

10.2 A middle-aged man with a varied occupational history presents with finger clubbing, fine inspiratory crepitations and central cyanosis. The chest radiograph reveals predominantly lower zone reticular nodular shadowing. Which ONE of the following disorders is the most likely explanation?
A Silicosis
B Sarcoidosis
C Asbestosis
D Ankylosing spondylitis
E Tuberculosis

10.3 A retired coal miner complains of increasing shortness of breath and a cough, occasionally productive of black sputum. Pulmonary function tests show an FEV1/FVC ratio of 0.5. A chest radiograph reveals multiple, large, coalescing, rounded opacities in the upper zones with some lesions showing cavitation. Which ONE of the following disorders is the most likely explanation?
A Bronchial carcinoma
B Cryptogenic fibrosing alveolitis
C Progressive massive fibrosis
D Emphysema
E Simple pneumoconiosis

10.4 Which ONE of the following features in a patient with pulmonary sarcoidosis is most likely to be associated with a good prognosis?
A Black ethnic origin
B Onset of disease in middle age
C Skin involvement
D Bone involvement
E Presentation with erythema nodosum and hilar lymphadenopathy

10.5 Which ONE of the following features suggests an alternative diagnosis to that of the adult respiratory distress syndrome?
A Hypoxaemia
B Reduced lung compliance
C Pulmonary capillary wedge pressure >18 mmHg
D Pulmonary hypertension
E High protein pulmonary oedema

10.6 A 60-year-old woman presenting with breathlessness and abdominal distension is found to have bilateral pleural effusions. Analysis of the pleural fluid reveals no evidence of bacteria and a protein concentration 15 g/L and lactic dehydrogenase concentration 150 iu/L. Which ONE of the following disorders is the most likely diagnosis?
A Myxoedema
B Pancreatitis
C Acute viral infection
D Polyarteritis nodosum
E Subphrenic abscess

10.7 A 66-year-old smoker presents with a history of weight loss and cough. Clinical examination revealed finger clubbing but no evidence of lymphadenopathy. The chest X-ray showed a cavitating mass in the right mid-zone. Which ONE of the following disorders is the most likely diagnosis?
A Squamous cell carcinoma
B Small cell carcinoma
C Adenocarcinoma
D Large cell carcinoma
E Carcinoid tumour

10.8 A 24-year-old plumber presents with a 10 day history of a non-productive cough, fever, anorexia and diarrhoea. Clinical examination reveals coarse crepitations at the right base and the chest X-ray shows patchy consolidation at the right base. The blood count is reported as showing red cell agglutination with a total white cell count 6.3×10^9/L, and platelet count 560×10^9/L. Which ONE of the following infectious organisms is the most likely cause?
A *Pneumocystis carinii*
B *Myocobacterium tuberculosis*
C *Mycoplasma pneumoniae*
D *Legionella pneumophila*
E *Klebsiella pneumoniae*

10.9 A 45 year-old woman is admitted to hospital having been found breathless and confused. Clinical examination showed evidence of central cyanosis, marked respiratory distress and a respiratory rate 36/minute. The following arterial blood gas results were obtained with the patient breathing air: pH 7.40, PaO_2 6.2 kPa and $PaCO_2$ 5.5 kPa. Which ONE of the following diagnoses is the likeliest explanation?

A Diabetic ketoacidosis
B Heroin overdose
C Motor neurone disease
D Asthma
E Anaemia

10.10 A 38-year-old, lifelong non-smoker complains of poor exercise tolerance and shortness of breath. He denied any problems with cough, sputum production or wheeze but on closer questioning, admitted to a non-productive cough most mornings especially during the winter months over the previous 5 years. Clinical examination revealed the absence of central cyanosis, poor but symmetrical chest expansion, cricosternal distance 2 cm after full inspiration, intercostal muscle indrawing and no added sounds on auscultation. Which ONE of the following features indicates the likeliest diagnosis?

A History of severe whooping cough in childhood
B Employment in the coal mining industry for 5 years
C Strong family history of premature ischaemic heart disease
D Alpha$_1$-antitrypsin phenotype PiZZ
E Occupational exposure to asbestos

10.11 A patient with a history of deteriorating exercise capacity is found to have cystic fibrosis. Clinical and laboratory investigations have confirmed central cyanosis, pulmonary hypertension and an FEV_1<25% predicted. Which ONE of the following features precludes the possibility of lung transplantation?

A A previous pleurodesis for recurrent pneumothorax
B Insulin dependent diabetes
C Steroid dependence
D Age 45
E Chronic bronchopulmonary aspergillosis

10.12 A 50-year-old woman and lifelong non-smoker presents with an intermittent wheeze associated with exertional breathlessness. There is no past history or family history of asthma, eczema or hay fever. The chest X-ray was normal. Which ONE of the following tests would be of most diagnostic value?

A Plethysmography

B Change in the forced expiratory volume following nebulized salbutamol

C Measurement of the transfer factor for carbon monoxide (TCO)

D The 6-minute walking test

E Arterial blood gas analysis

10.13 A 45-year-old male presents with breathlessness associated with a pleural effusion and a symmetrical, small-joint polyarthritis. Which ONE of the following findings MOST suggests an alternative diagnosis to rheumatoid arthritis?

A Subcutaneous nodules at the elbows

B Pericardial friction rub

C Positive anti-nuclear antibody test

D Onycholysis

E Fibrosing alveolitis

10.14 A 27-year-old male smoker presents with shortness of breath, cough and haemoptysis but is otherwise well. Pulmonary function tests (FEV/FVC) are normal and chest radiography reveals patchy consolidation in the mid- and lower zones. Urine analysis shows moderate proteinuria and haematuria but no red-cell casts. Which ONE of the following results of investigations is the most likely to be found?

A Positive anti-neutrophil cytoplasmic antibodies (ANCA)

B Normal transfer factor (TCO)

C Positive anti-basement membrane antibodies

D Normal histology on renal biopsy

E Anti-Ro and anti-La (SS-A and SS-B) antibodies

10.15 In a 39-year-old patient with chronic nasal polyps and exercise-induced asthma, exposure to which ONE of the following agents is most likely to precipitate an asthmatic attack?

A Ipratropium bromide

B Terbutaline

C Ibuprofen

D Combined contraceptive pill

E Trimethoprim

10.16 A young, healthy man moves from sea level to live in the mountains at an altitude of 4000 metres. Which ONE of the following physiological changes is MOST likely to occur?
A   Decrease in the $PaCO_2$
B   Decrease in plasma 2,3-diphosphoglycerate
C   Decrease in the minute ventilation
D   Decrease in the renal tubular bicarbonate excretion
E   Decrease in blood haemoglobin concentration

10.17 Electromyographic analysis of the muscles of the thorax is undertaken during deep inspiration to assess muscle activity. Which ONE of the following muscle groups is the likeliest to be INACTIVE?
A   Diaphragm
B   Internal intercostal muscles
C   External intercostal muscles
D   Sternomastoid muscle
E   Scalenus anterior muscle

10.18 A 41-year-old woman is referred to the medical outpatient department with pain and stiffness of the ankles and wrists, associated with a fever and painful red nodules over the shins. She was a heavy smoker who 2 weeks previously had been prescribed clarithromycin for an upper respiratory tract infection. Clinical examination revealed no evidence of finger clubbing, swollen ankles and a painful nodular rash affecting the lower limbs. Which ONE of the following disorders is the most likely diagnosis?
A   Sarcoidosis
B   Stevens–Johnson syndrome
C   Bronchial carcinoma
D   Wegener's granulomatosis
E   Severe acute respiratory syndrome (SARS)

10.19 A 28-year-old man presents with shortness of breath associated with bilateral pleural effusions and hilar lymphadenopathy on chest X-ray. A diagnostic pleural tap shows the fluid to be opalescent and milky. The plasma triglyceride concentration is reported as normal. Which ONE of the following disorders is the most likely diagnosis?
A   Bronchial carcinoma
B   Gorham's syndrome
C   Sarcoidosis
D   Systemic vasculitis
E   Lymphoma

10.20 A 35-year-old farmer living in Scotland develops breathlessness associated with an intermittent wheeze which responded to inhaled salbutamol. The peripheral white cell count (WBC) was increased at 18×10^9/L and the differential WBC indicated 20% eosinophils. The chest X-ray revealed diffuse, patchy pulmonary infiltrates. Which ONE of the following micro-organisms is the most likely to be responsible?

A *Aspergillus fumigatus*
B *Ascaris lumbricoides*
C *Mycoplasma pneumoniae*
D *Mycobacterium tuberculosis*
E *Micropolyspora faeni*

10.21 A 34-year-old man presents with exertional breathlessness of several months' duration. Clinical examination of the chest was normal but the chest X-ray showed diffuse reticular-nodular shadowing in both lower zones. Fluid obtained at broncho-alveolar lavage is reported to contain a marked increase in T and B lymphocytes, a reduced number of macrophages and without eosinophils. Which ONE of the following diagnoses is the most likely to explain the clinical picture?

A Chronic obstructive pulmonary disease
B Cryptogenic fibrosing alveolitis
C Extrinsic allergic alveolitis
D Asbestosis
E Sarcoidosis

10.22 Which ONE of the following statements about the normal pulmonary circulation is TRUE?

A Pulmonary veins drain blood from both pulmonary and bronchial arteries
B The azygous vein drains into the left atrium directly
C The pulmonary artery supplies the capillary bed in the bronchial walls
D The pulmonary arterioles dilate in response to hypoxia
E In the erect position the upper zones are more perfused than the mid- or lower zones

10.23 In which ONE of the following conditions would alveolar hypoventilation be an UNEXPECTED finding?

A Morbid obesity
B Diazepam overdose
C Myasthenia gravis
D Kyphoscoliosis
E Pulmonary oedema

10.24 Which ONE of the following results on pulmonary function tests would be the MOST likely to be found in a patient with severe emphysema?
A   Normal functional residual capacity (FRC)
B   Normal FEV$_1$
C   Normal FEV$_1$/FVC ratio
D   Raised RV/TLC ratio
E   Increased TCO

10.25 A lateral chest X-ray reveals a mass posteriorly overlying the spine. Which ONE of the following disorders is the MOST likely cause?
A   Thymoma
B   Tuberculous abscess
C   Pericardial cyst
D   Bronchogenic cyst
E   Teratoma

10.26 In which ONE of the following disorders would fine miliary calcification on chest X-ray be an expected finding?
A   Histoplasmosis
B   Asbestosis
C   Berylliosis
D   Sarcoidosis
E   Silicosis

10.27 Which ONE of the following statements about the phrenic nerve is TRUE?
A   It is derived from C6 and C7 spinal roots
B   It contains only motor fibres
C   On the left, it lies anterior to the aortic arch
D   When paralysed, it causes the affected hemidiaphragm to descend on sniffing
E   The left phrenic nerve passes through the central tendon of the diaphragm

10.28 During an attack of moderately severe asthma, which ONE of the following abnormalities in pulmonary function is the MOST likely to be found?
A   Decreased arterial PaO$_2$
B   Increased arterial PaCO$_2$
C   Decreased functional residual capacity (FRC)
D   Raised serum bicarbonate concentration
E   A normal peak expiratory flow rate (PEFR)

10.29 Which ONE of the following findings in a patient with cor pulmonale due to chronic obstructive pulmonary disease suggests an alternative or additional diagnosis?
A   Ascites
B   Tricuspid incompetence
C   Left bundle branch block on ECG
D   Right ventricular hypertrophy on echocardiography
E   Enlargement of hilar shadows on chest X-ray

10.30 Which ONE of the following findings in a patient with bronchial carcinoma is LEAST likely to be attributable to an unrelated, coexisting disorder?
A   Alopecia totalis
B   Hyponatraemia
C   Hypokalaemic alkalosis
D   Sensory neuropathy
E   Arthropathy

10.31 Which ONE of the following statements about BCG innoculation is TRUE?
A   A heat-killed strain of *Mycobacterium tuberculosis* is used
B   Protection efficacy rates should exceed 95%
C   Protection against leprosy is conferred
D   Regional lymphadenitis post-innoculation is best treated with isoniazid
E   All tuberculin-negative children should be inoculated at 2 years of age

10.32 Which ONE of the following findings in a patient with acute miliary tuberculosis suggests that an alternative or additional diagnosis is likely?
A   Normal chest X-ray
B   Negative tuberculin test
C   Aplastic anaemia
D   Splenomegaly
E   Haemoptysis

10.33 A patient with post-primary pulmonary tuberculosis is treated with rifampicin, pyrazinamide, ethambutol and isoniazid. Which ONE of the following adverse drug effects is LEAST likely to be attributable to rifampicin therapy?
A   Optic neuropathy
B   Discolouration of contact lenses
C   Deranged liver function tests
D   Decreased effectiveness of warfarin therapy
E   Haemolytic anaemia

10.34 Which ONE of the following effects is LEAST LIKELY to be attributable to positive end-expiratory pressure (PEEP) in the treatment of the adult respiratory distress syndrome (ARDS)?
A   A fall in functional residual capacity (FRC)
B   An increased oxygen saturation in the arteries
C   The prevention or delay of oxygen-induced lung damage
D   A fall in cardiac output
E   The risk of pulmonary barotrauma

10.35 Which ONE of the following features is MOST consistent with the diagnosis of primary pulmonary hypertension
A   Angina pectoris
B   Raised $PaCO_2$
C   Early diastolic murmur which is louder on expiration
D   Cannon in the jugular venous pulse
E   Inverted P waves on ECG

10.36 Which ONE of the following findings in a patient with idiopathic pulmonary haemosiderosis suggests an alternative or additional diagnosis?
A   History of recurrent haemoptysis
B   Onset under the age of 40 years
C   Presence of a hypochromic anaemia
D   Development of pulmonary fibrosis
E   Good response to desferrioxamine therapy

10.37 Which ONE of the following statements about hypertrophic pulmonary osteo-arthropathy (HPOA) is TRUE?
A   It may occur in the absence of finger clubbing
B   It is a recognized feature of benign pleural fibromas
C   It typically affects the large joints and spine
D   It is often associated with small-cell carcinoma of the bronchus
E   It is unlikely to resolve following tumour resection

10.38 Which ONE of the following statements about pulmonary function tests is TRUE?
A   Over 85% of the vital capacity can be expelled in one second in health
B   The transfer factor is measured using radio-labelled oxygen
C   The residual volume is decreased in chronic bronchitis and emphysema
D   The FEV/FVC ratio is typically normal in ankylosing spondylitis
E   Peak expiratory flow rates accurately reflect the severity of restrictive lung disease

10.39 Which ONE of the following statements about oxygen therapy is TRUE?

A At sea level, the partial pressure of oxygen in inspired air is 40 kPa

B Chronic domiciliary oxygen therapy is indicated only when pO_2 <6 kPa

C Dissolved oxygen does not contribute to tissue oxygenation in anaemia

D Oxygen toxicity in adults can produce retrolental fibroplasia

E Cyanosis unresponsive to 100% oxygen indicates right-to-left shunting >20%

10.40 In the delivery of oxygen therapy, which ONE of the following statements is TRUE?

A Inspired PaO_2 should not exceed 24% in patients with chronic ventilatory failure

B Venturi masks prevent the re-breathing of carbon dioxide

C Nasal cannulae deliver inspired oxygen concentration of 24% at 4 L/min

D Ventimasks require the oxygen to be humidified by passage through water

E Oxygen toxicity does not occur until after more than 72 hours of oxygen concentrations >40%

ANSWERS

10.1　A　✘　Reduced transfer factor
　　　B　✔　Any hyperkinetic state is likely to increase the transfer
　　　　　　factor
　　　C　✘　Reduced transfer factor
　　　D　✘　Reduced TCO as a result of less haemoglobin to bind CO
　　　E　✘　Normal or reduced transfer factor

10.2　A　✘
　　　B　✘
　　　C　✔　The remainder predominantly cause upper zone changes
　　　D　✘
　　　E　✘

10.3　A　✘
　　　B　✘
　　　C　✔　Upper zone involvement with cavitating lesions means
　　　　　　PMF
　　　D　✘
　　　E　✘

10.4　A　✘
　　　B　✘　Associated with an insidious onset and progressive
　　　　　　fibrosis
　　　C　✘
　　　D　✘
　　　E　✔　Subacute presentation in young white females typically
　　　　　　undergoes complete spontaneous remission within 2
　　　　　　years

10.5　A　✘
　　　B　✘
　　　C　✔　The wedge pressure should be less than 18 mmHg
　　　D　✘
　　　E　✘

10.6　A　✔　Transudate; consider cardiac failure, nephrotic syndrome
　　　　　　and cirrhosis
　　　B　✘
　　　C　✘　Usually pleural exudate (protein >30 g/L, LDH >200 iu/L)
　　　D　✘
　　　E　✘

10.7　A　✔　35% of lung malignancies and the most likely to cavitate
　　　B　✘　Rarely causes finger clubbing, unlike other lung tumours
　　　C　✘
　　　D　✘
　　　E　✘　Least common and rarely causes finger clubbing

10.8   A   ✗
      B   ✗
      C   ✔   Normal WBC and extra-pulmonary symptoms suggest atypical pneumonia
      D   ✗
      E   ✗

10.9   A   ✗   Absence of acidosis
      B   ✗   Usually hypoventilation with ventilatory failure
      C   ✗   Typically hypoventilation
      D   ✔   When severe, wheeze may be modest
      E   ✗   Causes features of chronic hypoxaemia

10.10   A   ✗   Not the features of bronchiectasis
      B   ✗   Too soon to develop symptomatic pneumoconiosis
      C   ✗   Unlikely to be relevant in the absence of exertional chest pain
      D   ✔   Homozygous alpha$_1$-antitrypsin deficiency, (protease inhibitor Pi)
      E   ✗

10.11   A   ✗
      B   ✗   Relative contraindications
      C   ✗
      D   ✗
      E   ✔   Absolute contraindications also include HIV infection, malignancy, irreversible organ failure and widespread vascular disease

---

10.12   A   ✗
      B   ✔   Diagnosis is asthma diagnosed by the reversibility of airways obstruction
      C   ✗
      D   ✗
      E   ✗

10.13   A   ✔   Always associated with rheumatoid factor antibodies
      B   ✗
      C   ✗   Commonly found in sero-positive RA
      D   ✗   Commoner in males
      E   ✗   Or bronchiolitis obliterans

10.14   A   ✗   Suggests Wegener's granulomatosis
      B   ✗   Often increased TCO associated with alveolar haemorrhage
      C   ✔ Goodpasture's syndrome with alveolar and glomerular disease
      D   ✗   IgG antibodies on the glomerular basement membrane
      E   ✗   Suggests primary Sjögren's syndrome

10.15 A ✗
B ✗
C ✔ Intrinsic asthma with sensitivity to aspirin and other NSAIDs
D ✗
E ✗

10.16 A ✔ Due to an increased ventilatory drive associated with hypoxia
B ✗ Increased 2,3 DPG reducing the affinity of Hb for oxygen
C ✗ Increased respiratory rate
D ✗ Increases to maintain a normal blood pH
E ✗ Increased erythropoietin production resulting in polycythaemia

10.17 A ✗
B ✔ Expiratory muscles
C ✗
D ✗
E ✗

10.18 A ✔ Typical presentation with arthralgia and erythema nodosum
B ✗ Usually a severe dermatitis with mucosal involvement
C ✗ HPOA does not occur in the absence of finger clubbing
D ✗
E ✗

10.19 A ✗ Rare at this age but could result in a chylothorax
B ✗ Benign lymphangiomas and haemangiomas of bone; produces osteolytic lesions and a chylothorax without lymphadenopathy
C ✗
D ✗
E ✔ Commonest cause of a chylous effusion

10.20 A ✔ Typical picture of acute allergic bronchopulmonary aspergillosis
B ✗ Rare but could produce an identical clinical picture
C ✗
D ✗
E ✗ Causes an allergic alveolitis — Farmer's lung

10.21 A ✗ Usually normal BAL cell count
B ✗ Increased neutrophils only on BAL
C ✗ Increased T cells, eosinophils and neutrophils on BAL
D ✗
E ✔

10.22   A   ✔
      B   ✗   The azygous vein drains into the superior vena cava
      C   ✗   Pulmonary arteries supply alveolar capillaries; bronchial arteries supply the bronchial and bronchiolar walls
      D   ✗   Hypoxia and acidosis cause pulmonary arterial constriction
      E   ✗   Gravity influences blood flow within the lung

10.23   A   ✗   Reduced alveolar ventilation may be due to maldistribution of inspired air, respiratory centre failure or reduced chest wall expansion
      B   ✗
      C   ✗
      D   ✗
      E   ✔   Hysteria and pulmonary oedema both cause hyperventilation

10.24   A   ✗   Emphysema is an obstructive disorder with low FEV_1/FVC ratio and raised FRC and RV/TLC ratio
      B   ✗   Reduced FEV_1
      C   ✗   Reduced FEV_1/FVC ratio
      D   ✔
      E   ✗   The alveolar surface area and both the TCO and KCO are reduced

10.25   A   ✗   The thymus lies anteriorly
      B   ✔   TB abscesses may arise from the vertebrae
      C   ✗   Pericardial cysts occur at the anterior cardiophrenic angle
      D   ✗   Bronchogenic cysts occur in the anterior and superior mediastinum
      E   ✗   Usually retrosternal space

10.26   A   ✔   Fine calcification on CXR can follow chickenpox and histoplasmosis
      B   ✗   Diffuse fibrosis and pleural plaques
      C   ✗
      D   ✗   Bilateral hilar lymphadenopathy, pulmonary infiltrates, miliary mottling
      E   ✗   'Egg-shell' calcification of enlarged hilar lymph nodes

10.27   A   ✗   The phrenic nerve is derived from C3–5; mainly C4
      B   ✗   Some afferent fibres, hence referred diaphragmatic pain
      C   ✔
      D   ✗   Hemidiaphragm is elevated and moves paradoxically during respiration
      E   ✗   The right nerve passes through the central tendon

10.28 A ✔ FEV$_1$ and PEFR fall and FRC rises due to 'air trapping'; arterial PaO$_2$ is reduced but PaCO$_2$ usually remains low or normal unless very severe
   B ✘
   C ✘
   D ✘ Metabolic acidosis may occur in children with acute asthma
   E ✘ PEFR falls

10.29 A ✘ With peripheral oedema and raised JVP
   B ✘
   C ✔ RBBB may be seen on ECG
   D ✘ Pulmonary hypertension
   E ✘ Secondary to pulmonary arterial hypertension

10.30 A ✔
   B ✘ Due to SIADH
   C ✘ Ectopic ACTH secretion produces hypokalaemic alkalosis
   D ✘ Carcinomatous neuropathy
   E ✘ Hypertrophic osteoarthropathy is usually due to squamous carcinoma, not small-cell carcinoma

10.31 A ✘ Attenuated live strains of *Mycobacterium bovis*
   B ✘ Variable protection rates of 0–84% but good protection against human and bovine TB and leprosy
   C ✔ *Mycobacterium leprae*
   D ✘ Ulceration of the wound and regional adenitis are common
   E ✘ It is offered mainly to subjects in high-risk groups

10.32 A ✘ Tubercles may be too small to be seen on X-ray
   B ✘ Ill patients may have tuberculin anergy
   C ✘ Splenomegaly and aplastic anaemia disappear with treatment
   D ✘
   E ✔ E.g. post-primary cavitating pulmonary TB

10.33 A ✔ Ethambutol produces optic neuropathy; isoniazid produces peripheral neuropathy due to pyridoxine deficiency
   B ✘ Tears often appear orange and this may stain some soft lenses
   C ✘
   D ✘ Increased metabolism of corticosteroids, contraceptives and warfarin
   E ✘ Causes hepatocellular not haemolytic jaundice

10.34 A ✔ Raises FRC to improve oxygen saturation
B ✘
C ✘ Allows ventilation with lower concentrations of oxygen to minimize oxygen-induced damage
D ✘
E ✘

10.35 A ✔ Severe dyspnoea, syncopal attacks and angina
B ✘ Hyperventilation and low $PaCO_2$
C ✘ The early diastolic murmur of Graham Steell fades on expiration
D ✘ Giant 'a' waves are a finding
E ✘

10.36 A ✘ A rare disease in young adults, characterized by recurrent haemoptysis, pulmonary X-ray shadowing and hypochromic anaemia
B ✘
C ✘ Typical
D ✘ Mediastinal lymphadenopathy can also occur
E ✔ Blood transfusion when necessary is the only supportive treatment

10.37 A ✘
B ✔
C ✘ Joint stiffness and pain in the long bones (wrists, ankles and knees)
D ✘ Typically with squamous-cell BUT NOT small-cell bronchial tumours
E ✘ Often improves; also can regress post-vagotomy

10.38 A ✘ More than 70% is normal
B ✘ Carbon monoxide is used
C ✘ Increased RV as the lungs are hyperinflated
D ✔ A restrictive disorder may develop
E ✘ A better measure of the severity of obstructive lung disorders

10.39 A ✘ PO_2 of inspired air = 20 kPa and declines with altitude
B ✘ Indicated when pO_2 <7.3 breathing air
C ✘ It does, especially when Hb is maximally saturated
D ✘ Occurs only in neonates
E ✔ Such shunts may be extra- or intra-pulmonary

10.40 A ✘ Patients on higher oxygen concentrations should be monitored
B ✔ Aids controlled delivery of oxygen concentrations <30%
C ✘ 30% at 2 L/min; useful for controlled oxygen therapy
D ✘ Humidification is only required with high concentration masks
E ✘ Can occur after >24 hours of >40% oxygen

11

Rheumatology

QUESTIONS

11.1 Which ONE of the following statements about articular cartilage is TRUE?
A   Composed of chondrocytes
B   Extremely vascular
C   Dependent on constant chondrocyte cell division for its repair
D   Highly innervated
E   Rich in the proteoglycans

11.2 Which ONE of the following statements about synovial membrane is TRUE?
A   Is composed principally of epithelial cells
B   Secretes synovial fluid from the stellate cells of the intercellular matrix
C   Receives its rich blood supply from adjacent cartilage
D   Is rich in unmedullated nerve fibres
E   Has an intercellular matrix containing hyaluronan, chondroitin sulphate and tenascin

11.3 Which ONE of the following statements about the structure of bone is TRUE?
A   Bone remodelling involves 50% of the bone surface in healthy adults each day
B   Cortical bone predominates in the epiphyses
C   Bone matrix is mainly composed of type I collagen
D   Trabecular bone is composed of Haversian systems
E   The lamellae of cortical bone run parallel to the surface of the bone

11.4 In measuring the bone density, which ONE of the following statements is TRUE?
A   Conventional X-rays of the skeleton will detect early changes in bone mineral density
B   DEXA bone densitometry is associated with a radiation dose similar to that of a chest X-ray
C   Bone mineral densitometry (BMD) is measured in grams of calcium per centimetre^2
D   The T-score expresses the number of standard deviations by which a patient's measurement differs from age and sex matched control subjects
E   The Z-score expresses the number of standard deviations by which a patient's measurement differs from healthy young control subjects

11.5   Which ONE of the following autoantibodies is associated with the following diseases?

A   Antinuclear antibodies — enteropathic arthritis

B   Anti-topoisomerase 1 antibodies — progressive systemic sclerosis (PSS)

C   Anti-SSA (anti-Ro) antibodies — systemic inflammatory response syndrome

D   Anti-centromere antibodies — Sneddon's syndrome

E   Antinuclear cytoplasmic antibodies — dermatomyositis

11.6   Which ONE of the following statements about antinuclear antibodies (ANA) is TRUE?

A   ANA are present in 50% of patients with systemic lupus erythematosus (SLE)

B   Single-stranded anti-DNA antibodies are specific to systemic lupus erythematosus

C   ANA persist at titres which are unrelated to clinical disease activity

D   Low titres of ANA are found in healthy subjects

E   ANA are characteristically present in high titres in patients with polyarteritis nodosa

11.7   A 25-year-old presents with an acute swelling of the right knee joint, pyrexia and night sweats of several days duration. Which ONE of the following statements is MOST consistent with the diagnosis of gonococcaemia?

A   Clinical features are more likely to occur in males than females

B   Tenosynovitis is likely to occur

C   Joint involvement is flitting rather than additive

D   Culture of the synovial fluid is likely to grow gonococci

E   The development of erythema nodosum is likely

11.8   In the investigation of a 50-year-old man with recent-onset low back pain, which ONE of the following statements is TRUE?

A   X-ray changes of spina bifida occulta would explain the symptom

B   Loss of lumbar lordosis suggests neoplastic vertebral infiltration

C   Exacerbation of pain with exercise suggests sacroiliitis

D   Myelography is the preferred investigation if neurological features develop

E   Spontaneous resolution within 12 weeks of onset occurs in the minority

11.9 **Which ONE of the following statements about patients with shoulder pain is TRUE?**
A Unlike infraspinatus tendonitis, supraspinatus tendonitis is associated with a 'painful arc'
B Bicipital tendinitis is associated with a painful arc
C Shoulder pain developing beyond 90° abduction suggests infraspinatus tendinitis
D Shoulder pain in all directions of movement suggests capsulitis
E Subscapularis tendinitis is suggested by pain worsening on resisted abduction

11.10 **Which ONE of the following statements about diffuse idiopathic skeletal hyperostosis (DISH) is TRUE?**
A Ossification along the anterolateral aspect of at least four contiguous vertebrae is likely
B The condition has a peak prevalence in adolescents
C Excessive vitamin D intake is thought to be responsible for the condition
D There is an association with HLA B27
E Pain in the axial skeleton is characteristic

11.11 **In a 24-year-old presenting with polyarthralgia, the subsequent development of joint swelling is MOST consistent with which ONE of the following diagnoses?**
A Rubella
B Depression
C Hypothyroidism
D Osteomalacia
E Diabetes insipidus

11.12 **In which ONE of the following diagnoses would the development of joint pain and swelling merit investigation to exclude an additional and unrelated diagnosis responsible for the arthritis?**
A Lyme disease
B Acromegaly
C Chondrocalcinosis
D Chronic sarcoidosis
E Tularaemia

11.13 **Which ONE of the following statements about osteoarthritis is TRUE?**
A It is present radiologically in at least 80% of patients aged 65 years or more
B It is more likely to be more generalized and more severe in males than females
C It is best characterized by degeneration of cartilage and synovial inflammation
D It is associated with decreased collagen synthesis in the affected cartilage
E It is best managed with anti-inflammatory doses of NSAIDs

11.14 A 29-year-old woman presents with a 6-month history of progressive arthritis of the knees and the PIP joints of the fingers. Rheumatoid and antinuclear antibody tests are negative. Which ONE of the following clinical features suggests that the diagnosis is more likely to be rheumatoid arthritis than psoriatic arthritis?

A   Pitting of the nails
B   Acute anterior uveitis
C   Association with HLA-DR4
D   Symmetrical joint involvement
E   Involvement of the sacro-iliac joints

11.15 Which ONE of the following extra-articular manifestations suggests a diagnosis of seronegative spondyloarthritis rather than rheumatoid arthritis?

A   Cutaneous ulceration
B   Pleural effusion
C   Enthesitis
D   Peripheral neuropathy
E   Hypersplenism

11.16 Which ONE of the following pathological changes is MOST consistent with the diagnosis of rheumatoid arthritis?

A   Diffuse synovial infiltration with neutrophils
B   Increased synovial fluid complement concentration
C   Subcutaneous nodules with numerous giant cells
D   Generalized lymph node hypoplasia
E   Progression to bony or fibrous ankylosis

11.17 Which ONE of the following statements about juvenile idiopathic arthritis is TRUE?

A   Still's disease typically presents with an acute poyarthritis
B   Seropositive polyarthritis typically resembles adult rheumatoid arthritis
C   Oligoarthritis typically affects boys in whom chronic iritis is common
D   Enthesitis-related arthritis typically affects girls
E   Polyarthritis rather than oligoarthritis is the commoner pattern of involvement

11.18 Which ONE of the following haematological findings is MOST consistent with the diagnosis of systemic lupus erythematosus?

A   Leucocytosis and thrombocytosis
B   Prolongation of the clotting time
C   Circulating anti-DNA and rheumatoid factor antibodies in high titre
D   Elevated CH_{50}, C_3 and C_4 complement levels in peripheral blood
E   Elevated C-reactive protein levels

11.19 Which ONE of the following clinical features suggests an alternative diagnosis to that of mixed connective tissue disease?
A Raynaud's phenomenon
B Diffuse interstitial pulmonary fibrosis
C Anti-RNA antibodies in high titres
D Involvement of the central nervous system
E Increased serum creatine kinase concentration

11.20 A 48-year-old man presents with an acutely painful and swollen pinna of the ear sparing the tragus. The past medical history includes deafness and episodes of peripheral polyarthritis. Which ONE of the following clinical features suggests an alternative diagnosis to relapsing polychondritis?
A Conductive deafness
B Episcleritis
C Second-degree heart block
D Proliferative glomerulonephritis
E Autoimmune hepatitis

11.21 A 30-year-old man presents with low back pain associated with stiffness, particularly noticeable in the mornings. Which ONE of the following features MOST suggests a mechanical rather than inflammatory cause for low backache?
A Radiation of pain down the back of one leg to the ankle
B An elevated C reactive protein
C Tenderness on lateral compression of the pelvis
D Absence of any abnormal physical sign
E Stiffness which persists on exercise

11.22 Which ONE of the following features is MOST typical of the fibromyalgia syndrome?
A Elevation of the ESR
B Coexistent symptoms of nocturnal diarrhoea
C Symptoms of insomnia and tiredness
D Rapid, spontaneous resolution
E Musculoskeletal pain without local tenderness

11.23 Which ONE of the following statements about musculoskeletal pains is TRUE?
A In inflammatory arthritis, pain typically worsens throughout the day
B Ligamentous strain produces pain which is usually only felt on movement
C The pain of impacted fractures is invariably worse on movement
D Muscle pain is typically unaffected by isometric contraction
E In osteoarthrosis, pain is improved on resting

11.24 In a 50-year-old woman presenting with neck pain, which ONE of the following statements is TRUE?
A Aggravation by sneezing suggests cervical spondylosis
B Radiation to the occiput suggests cranial arteritis
C Bilateral arm parasthesiae suggests angina pectoris is a likely diagnosis
D Absence of other joint pains excludes a diagnosis of rheumatoid arthritis
E History of syncopal episodes suggests cervical spondylosis

11.25 Which ONE of the following statements about the thoracic spine is TRUE?
A It is the commonest site of symptomatic disc protrusion
B It is more mobile in rotation than flexion and extension
C Lordosis of the thoracic spine is a normal finding in health
D Straightening of the thoracic spine is common in spinal osteoporosis
E Scoliotic deformity is common in patients with a history of poliomyelitis

11.26 Which ONE of the following statements about rheumatoid arthritis is TRUE?
A Onset characteristically occurs before the age of 30 years
B The female–male ratio is about 3:1
C There is a strong association with HLA-B8 status
D Progression to bone and cartilage destruction is rare
E Sparing of joints of the pelvic and shoulder girdle is typical

11.27 Which ONE of the following features would be the LEAST LIKELY finding in a patient presenting with active rheumatoid arthritis?
A Fever and weight loss
B Normocytic anaemia
C Anterior uveitis
D Thrombocythaemia
E Generalized lymphadenopathy

11.28 Which ONE of the following statements about the treatment of rheumatoid arthritis is TRUE?
A Bed rest should be avoided because of the risk of bony ankylosis
B Splinting of the affected joints reduces pain and swelling
C Associated anaemia responds promptly to oral iron therapy
D Systemic corticosteroids are contraindicated
E Non-steroidal anti-inflammatory drugs retard disease progression

11.29 **Which ONE of the following features confers the BEST prognosis in the functional outcome of patients presenting with rheumatoid arthritis?**
A   An insidious rather than acute onset of rheumatoid arthritis
B   A positive rheumatoid factor antibody test
C   The presence of subcutaneous nodules
D   The presence of extra-articular manifestations
E   Onset with palindromic rheumatism

11.30 **A 50-year-old woman presents with recurrent conjunctivitis and dry mouth. Which ONE of the following features is LEAST CONSISTENT with the diagnosis of primary Sjögren's disease?**
A   An increased incidence of lymphoma
B   Dryness of the eyes, mouth and vagina
C   Reduced lacrimal secretion rate
D   A good response to gold therapy
E   A positive IgM rheumatoid factor

11.31 **A 27-year-old man presenting with back pain and stiffness has a strong family history of back pain in the male members of his family. On investigation, he has elevation of the ESR and serum C-reactive protein with negative ANA and rheumatoid factor antibody tests. Which ONE of the following features is LEAST CONSISTENT with a diagnosis of seronegative spondyloarthritis?**
A   The presence of an asymmetrical oligoarthritis
B   Involvement of the cartilaginous joints
C   Enthesitis of tendinous insertions
D   Evidence of episcleritis
E   The presence of a soft diastolic murmur at the left sternal edge

11.32 **Which ONE of the following statements about the treatment of ankylosing spondylitis is TRUE?**
A   Systemic corticosteroid therapy is contraindicated
B   Prolonged bed rest accelerates functional recovery
C   Spinal radiotherapy modifies the course of the disease
D   Spinal deformity usually progresses despite intensive physiotherapy
E   The presence of hip involvement confers a poorer prognosis

11.33 **Which ONE of the following statements about Reiter's disease is TRUE?**
A   Anterior uveitis develops more often than conjunctivitis
B   Sacro-iliitis and spondylitis develops in most patients
C   Small joint polyarthritis is typically symmetrical
D   Onset 1–3 weeks following bacterial dysentery
E   Arthritis typically resolves within 3–6 months of onset

11.34 **A 33-year-old man presents with pain and stiffness of the ankles and toes which is most marked on rising from bed in the morning. Clinical examination reveals the presence of scaly plaques suggesting psoriasis in the scalp. Which ONE of the following statements about psoriatic arthritis is TRUE?**
A   Joint involvement typically precedes the onset of psoriasis
B   Arthritis is likely to affect 25% of patients with psoriasis
C   Absence of psoriatic nail changes suggests that arthritis may not be due to psoriasis
D   The arthritis is likely to be very different to rheumatoid arthritis in its distribution
E   A good response to hydroxochloroquine is likely

11.35 **A 42-year-old Asian woman, resident in the UK for the previous 3 years, is referred to the outpatient clinic with tiredness, malaise and non-specific aches and pains. Clinical examination is unremarkable except for muscle weakness demonstrable as the patient rises from her chair. Biochemical investigations reveal a serum calcium 1.7 mmol/L, serum phosphate 0.7 mmol/L and normal liver function values other than an elevation of the serum alkaline phosphatase 210 iu/L. Which ONE of the following statements is TRUE?**
A   The proximal myopathy suggests that the likeliest diagnosis is thyrotoxicosis
B   Metabolic bone disease is characteristically painless
C   The plasma parathyroid hormone level is likely to be low
D   If renal disease is present, 25-hydroxycholecalciferol therapy is advisable
E   Pseudofractures are best detected using isotope bone scanning

ANSWERS

11.1   A   ✔   Plus a collagen framework which entraps proteoglycans
        B   ✘   Avascular
        C   ✘   Aggrecan proteoglycan synthesis rather than cell division
                is critical for repair
        D   ✘   Devoid of a nerve supply
        E   ✘   Especially aggrecan, a protein core with keratin and
                chondroitin sidechains

11.2   A   ✘   Macrophages and fibroblast-like cells
        B   ✘   Fluid is secreted by type B fibroblasts
        C   ✘   It provides the blood supply to the cartilage
        D   ✘   Devoid of a nerve supply
        E   ✔   Together with type VI collagen

11.3   A   ✘   Bone remodelling involves 10% of the bone surface in health
        B   ✘   Cortical bone predominates in the diaphyses and
                trabecular bone in the epiphyses
        C   ✔   Collagen fibrils are bonded by pyridinium cross-links
                increasing the tensile strength
        D   ✘   Cortical bone is composed of Haversian systems
        E   ✘   The lamellae of trabecular bone run parallel and cortical
                bone run concentrically

11.4   A   ✘   At least 30% of bone mineral needs to have been lost from
                the skeleton
        B   ✔   Similar to that of a chest X-ray; effective dose equivalent
                is about 20 microSieverts
        C   ✘   Grams of hydroxyapatite per centimetre^2
        D   ✘   The Z-score; osteoporotic patients typically have a low
                T score and low Z-score
        E   ✘   The T-score; osteopenia T-scores = −1 − −2.5; osteoporosis
                T-score <−2.5

11.5   A   ✘   Rheumatoid arthritis, SLE, progressive systemic sclerosis
                and autoimmune hepatitis
        B   ✔
        C   ✘   Sjögren's syndrome is associated with anti-SSA (anti-Ro)
                and anti-SSB (anti-La)
        D   ✘   CREST syndrome; Sneddon's syndrome is the
                antiphospholipid syndrome
        E   ✘   Associated with Wegener's granulomatosis and systemic
                vasculitis

11.6   A   ✘   Positive ANA is found in 95% of SLE patients
        B   ✘   High titres of double stranded anti-DNA antibodies are
                highly suggestive of SLE
        C   ✘   Rising titre may precede clinical deterioration
        D   ✔   Low titres are particularly often found in the elderly
        E   ✘   There are no auto-antibodies of diagnostic value in
                polyarteritis nodosa

11.7   A   ✗   Females > males; males tend to present with urethritis
      B   ✔   Tenosynovitis is a typical feature
      C   ✗   Usually additive joint involvement
      D   ✗   Positive synovial fluid culture in only 25%; check blood and genital tract cultures
      E   ✗   A sparse pustular rash is characteristic

11.8   A   ✗   Typically asymptomatic
      B   ✗   A non-specific finding in back pain of many causes
      C   ✗   Exercise typically ameliorates pain in sacroiliitis
      D   ✔   Magnetic resonance scanning is indicated if there are neurological features
      E   ✗   Only about 3% of cases persist for more than 3 months

11.9   A   ✗   Same 'painful arc' for both conditions
      B   ✗   The bicipital groove may be tender
      C   ✗   Suggests acromioclavicular joint disease
      D   ✔   'Frozen shoulder'
      E   ✗   Pain worsens on resisted internal rotation

11.10   A   ✔   Definitive radiological criteria
      B   ✗   In the elderly; Scheuermann's osteochondritis is typically seen in adolescence
      C   ✗   Caused by excessive proteoglycan synthesis at entheses
      D   ✗   Associated with NIDDM, gout, obesity and hypertension
      E   ✗   Typically absent, though heel pain and hypertrophic hip osteoarthrosis may occur

11.11   A   ✔   Especially in rubella in adults
      B   ✗   Causes muscle and joint pains but not arthritis
      C   ✗   Can cause muscle aches and pains
      D   ✗   Aches and pains are prominent in osteomalacia
      E   ✗

11.12   A   ✗   Relapsing pauciarticular large joint involvement
      B   ✗   Small and large joint involvement with hypertrophic spondylosis
      C   ✗   Pseudogout
      D   ✗   Small joint involvement
      E   ✔   Cutaneous ulceration and fever

11.13   A   ✔   Often symptomatic
      B   ✗   Females are more severely affected
      C   ✗   Synovial inflammation is mild; proliferation of new bone and cartilage is typical
      D   ✗   Collagen turnover is increased as total collagen declines
      E   ✗   Simple analgesics are equally effective and have fewer adverse effects

11.14 A ✗ And onycholysis are typical of psoriatic arthritis
       B ✗ Usually episcleritis and keratoconjunctivitis sicca in RA
       C ✔ Present in 50–75% of Caucasians with rheumatoid arthritis
       D ✗ May occur in both disorders
       E ✗ Affects large and small joints with relative sparing of spinal joints

11.15 A ✗ Vasculitis and ulceration of nodules is typical of RA
       B ✗ Typical of RA; fluid is an exudate not a transudate
       C ✔ Commonly at points of bony prominences, e.g. hips and iliac crest
       D ✗ Due to arteritis of the vasa nervorum in RA
       E ✗ Hypersplenism is rare in RA (Felty's syndrome)

11.16 A ✗ Infiltration with lymphocytes, especially CD4 T cells and plasma cells
       B ✗ CH50, C3 and C4 levels are low (activation of the classical pathway)
       C ✗ Characteristic feature is central fibrinoid necrosis
       D ✗ Generalized hyperplasia with non-tender lymphadenopathy
       E ✔

11.17 A ✗ Systemic features of illness predominate rather than arthritic features
       B ✔ Usually presents over the age of 8 years (10% of all juvenile polyarthritis)
       C ✗ Usually girls especially with positive ANA and asymptomatic chronic iritis
       D ✗ Boys > girls; 75% HLA-B27 positive and resembles ankylosing spondylitis
       E ✗ Oligoarticular disease predominates, i.e. four or fewer joints affected

11.18 A ✗ Leucopenia and thrombocytopenia are typical
       B ✗ Antiphospholipid syndrome is associated with a procoagulant effect
       C ✔ Positive tests in low titre are however common and diagnostically unhelpful
       D ✗ Depressed, suggesting activation of the classical complement pathway
       E ✗ Rarely elevated unless coincidental infection is present

11.19 A ✗ A common feature
       B ✗
       C ✗ Antibodies to extractable nuclear antigens (anti-ENA) are usually present
       D ✔ Similarly, cardiac and renal involvement are very rare
       E ✗ Proximal muscle weakness and tenderness with high serum CK and LDH

11.20   A   ✗   May produce conductive or sensorineural deafness and vestibular damage
      B   ✗   And scleritis, keratitis and uveitis
      C   ✗   A-V conduction defects due to small vessel vasculitis
      D   ✗   Focal, proliferative glomerulonephritis is associated with the condition
      E   ✔   Nasal chondritis and laryngeal involvement with hoarseness and stridor may occur

11.21   A   ✗   Suggests lumbar nerve root compression
      B   ✗   Suggests an active inflammatory pathology
      C   ✗   Suggests sacro-iliitis
      D   ✗   Occasionally, serious pathology can occur without physical signs
      E   ✔   Rest pain and stiffness which improve on exercise suggest inflammatory disease

11.22   A   ✗   High ESR suggests an inflammatory disorder
      B   ✗   Suggests an enteropathic arthritis
      C   ✔   And other psychosomatic disorders
      D   ✗   Often very chronic
      E   ✗   Multiple tender points are characteristic

11.23   A   ✗   Often improved by physical activity
      B   ✗   Continuous but aggravated by movement
      C   ✗   Loss of normal function may be the only feature
      D   ✗
      E   ✔   Typically aggravated by movement and relieved by rest

11.24   A   ✗   Suggests cervical disc prolapse; look for neurological signs
      B   ✗   Common in tension headache
      C   ✗   Suggest cervical radiculopathy
      D   ✗   RA typically involves atlanto-axial articulations
      E   ✔   Due to vertebral artery compression

11.25   A   ✗   Lumbar disc prolapse predominates
      B   ✗
      C   ✗
      D   ✗   Spine becomes kyphotic
      E   ✔   And also kyphoscoliosis

11.26   A   ✗   Age of onset follows a normal distribution (no age group is exempt)
      B   ✔   After the age of 55, affects 5% of women and 2% of men
      C   ✗   HLA-DR4 is found in 75% of affected individuals
      D   ✗   Bony ankylosis is the rule
      E   ✗   Large and small joints are affected

11.27 A ✗ Occurence with minimal joint symptoms makes the diagnosis difficult
       B ✗ Anaemia is classically normochromic and normocytic
       C ✔ Anterior uveitis is associated with the seronegative spondyloarthritis
       D ✗ Modest elevation in platelet count is common
       E ✗ More obvious in nodes draining actively inflamed joints

11.28 A ✗ Bed rest is of great value and without risk of bony ankylosis
       B ✔ Reduces joint pain and may reduce contractures
       C ✗ Not usually iron deficient and reflects disease activity
       D ✗ Steroids may also lessen the risk of disease progression
       E ✗ NSAIDs are not disease modifying drugs unlike gold, penicillamine and immunosuppressant agents

11.29 A ✗ An explosive onset confers a relatively better prognosis
       B ✗
       C ✗ Always strongly positive for rheumatoid factor
       D ✗
       E ✔ The presence of periods of remission is a favourable sign

11.30 A ✗
       B ✗
       C ✗ Best demonstrated using the Shirmer test
       D ✔ High incidence of drug allergies especially to gold and antibiotics
       E ✗ Occurs in over 80% but NOT diagnostic of primary Sjögren's disease

11.31 A ✗ Axial joints are usually involved initially; only 10% present with peripheral joint disease
       B ✗ Sacroiliac joint disease is rare in seropositive arthritides
       C ✗ Achilles tendonitis is common
       D ✔ Typically acute anterior uveitis; episcleritis suggests RA
       E ✗ Aortitis causing aortic regurgitation

11.32 A ✗ Can be invaluable and especially for acute iritis
       B ✗ In contrast to RA, the patient with AS stiffens with bed rest
       C ✗ Only used to improve symptoms
       D ✗ Education regarding appropriate back exercises is vital
       E ✔ As does extra articular disease

11.33 A ✗ Conjunctivitis is the classical ocular manifestation
       B ✗ Occurs in only 15% of patients
       C ✗ Arthritis is asymmetrical, involving large or small joints
       D ✔ Similar delay following sexually acquired infections
       E ✗ 10% of patients have chronic active arthritis 20 years after onset

11.34 A ✗ Occasionally there is no evidence of skin disease at onset
     B ✗ Occurs in around 7%
     C ✔ Pitting and onycholysis of the nails are characteristic
     D ✗ Most patients have a rheumatoid-like pattern of arthritis
     E ✗ Hydroxychloroquine may precipitate an exfoliative
       reaction

11.35 A ✗ The diagnosis is osteomalacia
     B ✗ Pain may be generalized and severe
     C ✗ Typically elevated in contrast to the low serum calcium
       level
     D ✗ 1alpha hydroxycholecalciferol since 1 alpha hydroxylation
       is impaired
     E ✔ 'Looser's zones' are translucent bands and can also be
       seen on X-ray

12

Psychiatry

QUESTIONS

12.1 An 80-year-old woman is found wandering the streets in her nightclothes in the early evening and is brought by the police to the casualty department. Which ONE of the following features would be the MOST useful in identifying dementia rather than an acute confusional state as the underlying problem?
A Impaired consciousness which varies over the following 12 hours
B Impaired attention span and ability to concentrate
C Impaired long-term memory with disorientation in time and place
D Illusions, hallucinations and delusions
E Psychomotor retardation with features of depression

12.2 Which ONE of the following clinical features is MOST likely to be found in association with intellectual impairment in an elderly patient presenting with acute confusion?
A Disordered thought content
B Auditory hallucination
C Inappropriate optimism
D Disorientation in time and place without short-term memory loss
E Impaired serial 7s test and loss of abstract thinking ability

12.3 Which ONE of the following definitions of psychological phenomena is TRUE?
A Delusions — abnormal perceptions of normal external stimuli
B Illusions — unreasonably persistent, firmly held false beliefs
C Hallucinations — normal perceptions provoked by external stimuli
D Depersonalization — normal perception of altered reality
E Phobia — obsessive repetition in an attempt to control anxiety

12.4 Which ONE of the following features is a cardinal element of behavioural therapy?
A Hypersensitization
B Avoidance of all stress
C Operant conditioning
D Exploration of repressed unpleasant experiences
E Modification of patterns of negative thinking

12.5 **Which ONE of the following features is a cardinal element of cognitive therapy?**
A Restructuring psychological conflicts and behaviour
B Identification of negative patterns of automatic thoughts
C Attempt to disconnect thoughts and mood from behaviour
D Review of childhood experiences and reassessment of personality development
E Transactional analysis

12.6 **Which ONE of the following statements about psychiatric drug treatments is TRUE?**
A Risperidone selectively blocks dopamine receptors more than serotonin receptors
B Antidepressant drug therapy directly blocks noradrenaline (norepinephrine) and serotonin neural secretion
C The adverse effects of tricyclic antidepressants result from their anticholinergic effects
D Monoamine oxidase inhibitors are more potent antidepressants than tricyclics
E Lithium carbonate inhibits catechol-O-methyl transferase to prevent recurrent depression

12.7 **Which ONE of the following statements about phenothiazine antipsychotic drug therapy is TRUE?**
A Phenothiazines block central nervous beta$_2$ receptors
B The onset of dystonia and dyskinesia are likely to be attributable to cholinergic side-effects
C Long-term ocular complications include corneal and lenticular opacities
D The onset of galactorrhoea suggests that the likeliest cause would be a hypothalamic tumour
E Patients commencing clozapine therapy should have regular monitoring of their renal function

12.8 **Which ONE of the following clinical features is MOST consistent with a diagnosis of a generalized anxiety disorder?**
A Feelings of worthlessness
B Loss of energy, libido and interest
C Excessive guilt
D Breathlessness and dizziness
E Claustrophobia and agoraphobia

12.9 **A 49-year-old labourer is admitted at 10 a.m. following a fall from scaffolding at work. He smells strongly of alcohol. Which ONE of the following MOST suggests chronic alcohol dependence?**
A Consumption of a wide range of alcoholic beverages
B Increasing tolerance of alcohol
C Nausea and retching in the morning
D Progressive weight loss
E Refractory constipation

12.10 In an elderly patient who becomes confused following admission to a medical ward, which ONE of the following MOST suggests an acute alcohol withdrawal state?
A Hypersomnia
B Visual or auditory hallucinations
C Impaired short-term memory
D Depression and morbid jealousy
E Nystagmus and ophthalmoplegia

12.11 Which ONE of the following clinical features is MOST consistent with a diagnosis of a benzodiazepine withdrawal state?
A Diminished sensory perception
B Hallucinations and delusions
C Ataxia and dementia
D Manic depressive-like disorder
E Poverty of ideas and speech

12.12 Which ONE of the following clinical features is MOST consistent with gastrointestinal disease rather than a somatization disorder?
A Multiple previous medical consultations for unexplained ill health
B Preoccupation with the possibility of physical illness
C Chronic abdominal pain as the sole symptom
D Diarrhoea and weight loss without abdominal pain
E Abnormal illness behaviour dating from childhood

12.13 In an adolescent female presenting with painless vomiting and weight loss, which ONE of the following features is MOST consistent with the diagnosis of anorexia nervosa?
A Dysmenorrhoea
B Buccal and skin crease pigmentation
C Weight <25% below the predicted norm
D Normal perception of body weight and image
E Retardation of physical sexual development

12.14 In an adolescent female presenting with painless vomiting, which ONE of the following features is MOST consistent with the diagnosis of bulimia nervosa?
A Onset of symptoms at puberty
B Dramatic weight loss
C Uncontrolled carbohydrate bingeing
D Vomiting before meals
E Compulsive desire to exercise

12.15 Following an apparently minor episode of self-poisoning, which ONE of the following factors is associated with a subsequent increased risk of suicide?
  A   Females rather than males
  B   Aged <25 years rather than aged >50 years
  C   Absence of a suicide note or previous suicide attempts
  D   Absence of previous physical or mental illness
  E   Living alone or recently separated from partner

12.16 Which ONE of the following factors suggests a psychiatric illness rather than an organic brain disorder?
  A   Symptom onset for the first time at the age of 55
  B   A family history of major psychiatric illness
  C   Absence of a previous history of psychiatric illness
  D   Absence of a precipitating adverse life event
  E   Episodes of dysphasia and impaired short-term memory

12.17 Which ONE of the following features suggests an obsessional disorder?
  A   Repetitive behaviour
  B   Attention-seeking behaviour
  C   Behaviour regarded as normal by the patient
  D   Behaviour that is not resisted by the patient
  E   Development of a depressive disorder

12.18 Which ONE of the following features best characterizes the early stages of schizophrenia?
  A   Early-morning waking
  B   Loss of emotional responses
  C   Visual hallucinations
  D   A feeling of depersonalization
  E   Failure to recall recent events

12.19 Which ONE of the following features is MOST consistent with the diagnosis of Korsakoff's psychosis?
  A   Impaired long-term memory
  B   Recent history of epileptic seizures
  C   Presence of a peripheral neuropathy
  D   The use of neologisms
  E   Occurrence of visual hallucinations

12.20 A 55-year-old man presents to his general practitioner with a 6-month history of insomnia, painless nausea, vomiting and diarrhoea. Which ONE of the following features is LEAST likely to relate to the diagnosis of a chronic alcohol dependency state?
  A   Depression
  B   Relief of withdrawal symptoms by alcohol ingestion
  C   Relapses even after prolonged abstinence
  D   Feelings of guilt about alcohol use
  E   Increased tolerance of alcohol

12.21 Which ONE of the following drugs is MOST likely to lead to chronic physical dependency when prescribed as long-term therapy?
A Temazepam
B Amitriptyline
C Paracetamol
D Naproxen
E Orlistat

12.22 A 22-year-old woman is referred by her general practitioner with dizziness and peripheral paraesthesiae. The past medical history includes numerous medically unexplained symptoms dating back to childhood. Which ONE of the following features is MOST in keeping with a diagnosis of a conversion disorder?
A An apparent lack of concern about her symptoms
B Early morning waking
C Feelings of depersonalization
D Manipulative behaviour
E Repeated hand-washing

12.23 An 80-year-old woman is referred to the outpatient department with a history of progressive behavioural problems associated with nominal dysphasia. Which ONE of the following features is INCONSISTENT with a diagnosis of Alzheimer's dementia?
A A family history of dementia
B An altered sleep pattern
C Bilateral extensor plantar responses
D Topographagnosia
E Dysarthria

12.24 Which ONE of the following features is MOST suggestive of a neurotic rather than psychotic disorder?
A Grandiose delusions
B Lack of insight and awareness of a problem
C Auditory hallucinations
D Cognitive impairment
E A monosymptomatic phobia with a family history of phobic disorder

12.25 Which ONE of the following features suggests an abnormal illness behaviour?
A A relentless search for an underlying disease
B An increased sense of responsibility for illness and its treatment
C A reluctance to adopt the sick role
D Disability which is consistent with the patient's signs and symptoms
E An obsession with health-promoting activities

12.26 Which ONE of the following features is LEAST CONSISTENT with the diagnosis of somatization disorder?
A Multiple, medically unexplained physical complaints
B Preoccupation with the fear of illness
C Onset of symptoms before the age of 30 years
D Previous history of unsuccessful surgical procedures
E Conscious simulation of illness to obtain exemption from work

12.27 Which ONE of the following features is LEAST characteristic of hypomania?
A Flight of ideas
B Rhyming speech
C Hypersomnia
D Weight gain
E Sexual promiscuity

12.28 In a patient with manic depression, which ONE of the following features would be LEAST likely to be due to an adverse drug effect from lithium carbonate therapy?
A An exacerbation of psoriasis
B A progressive tremor
C Polyuria resistant to vasopressin
D Development of a goitre
E Onset of thyrotoxicosis

12.29 A 30-year-old woman presents with features of a generalized anxiety disorder. Which ONE of the following differential diagnoses would be LEAST likely to explain her symptomatology?
A Alcohol withdrawal syndrome
B Thyrotoxicosis
C Hypoglycaemia
D Phaeochromocytoma
E Carcinoid syndrome

12.30 A 70-year-old retired university lecturer presents with anorexia, loss of interest in his previous hobbies and paranoid delusions. His condition deteriorates and following an attempt to hang himself, he is admitted to hospital for psychiatric evaluation. Which ONE of the following features is an indication for electroconvulsive therapy (ECT)?
A A previous history of alcohol withdrawal syndrome
B The recent finding of an elevated serum thyroxine and low plasma TSH
C Absence of a response to 4 weeks of antidepressant drug therapy
D Depression associated with a longstanding panic disorder
E Depressive stupor associated with nutritional difficulties

ANSWERS

12.1 A ✗ This suggests a confusional state, especially if fluctuant
      B ✗ Acutely confused patients may therefore find even simple mental arithmetic difficult
      C ✗ Suggests a confusional state
      D ✗ Such perceptual disturbances are common in confusion
      E ✔ Dementia may mimic depressive illness

12.2 A ✗ Suggests a psychotic disorder
      B ✗ Suggests a psychotic disorder
      C ✗ Suggests mania or hypomania
      D ✗ Suggests an acute confusional state
      E ✔ Impaired attention span in acute confusional state may also diminish these abilities

12.3 A ✗ Unreasonably persistent, firmly held false beliefs
      B ✗ Abnormal perceptions of normal external stimuli
      C ✗ Abnormal perceptions without external stimuli
      D ✔ Often with derealization
      E ✗ Abnormal fear leading to avoidance behaviour typical of a neurosis

12.4 A ✗ Systematic desensitization is used e.g. in the treatment of phobias
      B ✗ Exposure to maximal stress (flooding) can be useful
      C ✔ With positive and negative reinforcement
      D ✗ This is used in interpretative psychotherapy
      E ✗ Feature of cognitive therapy

12.5 A ✗ Undertaken in psychotherapy
      B ✔ Reassess the validity of negative thoughts and views and develop positive views
      C ✗ Awareness of connections between thoughts, mood and behaviour can alter behaviour
      D ✗ Used in psychotherapy
      E ✗ Form of psychotherapy

12.6 A ✗ Blocks $5HT_2$ receptors more than D_2 receptors (hence fewer parkinsonian features)
      B ✗ Blocks synaptic reuptake of noradrenaline (norepinephrine) and serotonin
      C ✔ Dry mouth, constipation, tachycardia, etc.
      D ✗ Less potent and with potentially more serious drug interactions
      E ✗ Inhibitor of neurotransmitter-induced phosphoinositide hydrolysis

12.7   A   ✘   Block CNS dopamine D_2 receptors hence the features of parkinsonism
      B   ✘   These side-effects are due to dopamine receptor blockade
      C   ✔   Chlorpromazine may also produce a *retinitis pigmentosa*-like syndome
      D   ✘   Like gynaecomastia, it is a typical side-effect of dopamine receptor blockade
      E   ✘   Neutropenia occurs in 3% and requires careful monitoring of the FBC

12.8   A   ✘   Suggests depression
      B   ✘   Suggests depression
      C   ✘   Suggests depression
      D   ✔   Typical somatic symptoms
      E   ✘   Suggests depression

12.9   A   ✘   Contraction of the drinking repertoire
      B   ✘   Decreasing tolerance
      C   ✔   Often relieved by alcohol
      D   ✘   Often weight gain (calorific value of alcohol 7 Kcal/gram)
      E   ✘   Diarrhoea

12.10   A   ✘   Early-morning waking with anxiety and tremor
      B   ✔   Typically persecutory if auditory
      C   ✘   Suggests Korsakoff psychosis
      D   ✘   Suggests alcohol dependence
      E   ✘   Suggests Wernicke's encephalopathy

12.11   A   ✘   Typically increased perception with depersonalization
      B   ✔   And other perceptual disorders
      C   ✘   Seizures may occur in acute withdrawal
      D   ✘   Affect is not typically disturbed
      E   ✘   Agitation rather than retardation

12.12   A   ✘   Psychological explanations are often firmly rejected
      B   ✘   Suggests a somatization disorder
      C   ✘   Pain as an isolated symptom is much more likely to be functional in origin
      D   ✔   Not a feature of the irritable bowel syndrome
      E   ✘   Suggests a somatization disorder

12.13   A   ✘   Amenorrhoea
      B   ✘   Suggests an endocrinopathy, e.g. hypoadrenalism
      C   ✔   In contrast to bulimia nervosa
      D   ✘   Emaciation is unrecognized by the patient
      E   ✘   And psychosexual retardation

12.14 A ✘ Typically post-pubertal
      B ✘ Body weight maintained
      C ✔
      D ✘ Self-induced vomiting after meals associated with dieting after binges
      E ✘ Suggests anorexia nervosa

12.15 A ✘ Greater risk in males
      B ✘ Greater risk in the older age groups
      C ✘ Suicide note often left and usually a history of previous attempts
      D ✘ Often also associated with drug or alcohol abuse
      E ✔ Or bereavement

12.16 A ✘ Suggests organic brain disease
      B ✔ Especially depressive illness
      C ✘ Favours organic brain disorder
      D ✘ Adverse life events commonly predate the onset of psychiatric illness
      E ✘ Strongly suggest organic brain syndrome

12.17 A ✔ Usually repetitive and regarded as abnormal by the patient; many patients are reluctant to talk about the problem
      B ✘
      C ✘
      D ✘
      E ✘ It can progress to depression

12.18 A ✘ Depression
      B ✔ Passivity phenomena are common
      C ✘ Hallucinations are usually auditory; visual hallucinations are uncommon
      D ✘ Suggests anxiety state
      E ✘ Dementia and organic brain syndromes

12.19 A ✘ Short-term memory impaired
      B ✘ Fits are usually a feature of alcohol withdrawal
      C ✔ 'Psychosis polyneuritica' in Korsakoff's original description
      D ✘
      E ✘ A feature of delirium tremens

12.20 A ✘ Increased suicide risk, especially in males
      B ✘
      C ✘
      D ✘
      E ✔ Tolerance is increased initially then rapidly decreases as the illness progresses

12.21 A ✔ Use should be limited to short-term only
B ✘ May be required long-term to prevent relapse
C ✘ Unlike all opiates which are potentially addictive
D ✘
E ✘ Lipase inhibitor

12.22 A ✔ 'Belle indifference'
B ✘ Suggests depression
C ✘ Suggests anxiety
D ✘
E ✘ Suggests an obsessive compulsive disorder

12.23 A ✘ The family history sometimes suggests an autosomal
dominance trait
B ✘ A common finding
C ✔ Organic brain syndromes must be excluded
D ✘ Inability to find one's way in familiar surroundings
E ✘

12.24 A ✘ Suggests manic disorder or GPI
B ✘ Psychosis
C ✘ Psychosis
D ✘
E ✔ Morbidity risk of 30% in first-degree relatives of patients
with panic disorder

12.25 A ✔
B ✘ Abrogation of all responsibility for illness to the doctors
C ✘
D ✘ Disability is disproportionate to the signs and symptoms
E ✘ Avoidance of health-promoting roles and activities

12.26 A ✘ Often arising from early childhood
B ✘ Hypochondriasis
C ✘ Most uncommon presenting after the age of 30 years
D ✘ Characteristic; especially appendicectomy and
hysterectomy
E ✔ This suggests malingering

12.27 A ✘
B ✘
C ✔ Patients are typically restless, quick-witted, self-confident
and need little sleep
D ✘ May lose weight because they are too distracted to eat
E ✘

12.28 A ✘ Psoriasis may be exacerbated
B ✘ Also nausea, anorexia, and diarrhoea
C ✘ Produces nephrogenic diabetes insipidus
D ✘
E ✔ Inhibits thyroidal release of T_4 to produce hypothyroidism

12.29 A ✗ Typical features of anxiety
B ✗ Simulates anxiety states
C ✗ Simulates anxiety states
D ✗ Excess adrenaline (epinephrine) and noradrenaline (norepinephrine) secretion
E ✔ Flushing, wheezing and diarrhoea

12.30 A ✗
B ✗ Suggests thyrotoxicosis
C ✗ Response to antidepressant therapy may be delayed for 12 weeks
D ✗
E ✔ May need the appointment of a legal guardian

13

Dermatology

QUESTIONS

13.1 Which ONE of the following clinical features of a pigmented skin lesion MOST suggests a benign rather than a malignant melanoma?
A Symmetrical macule
B Irregular border
C Irregular colour
D Diameter >0.5 cm
E Irregular elevation

13.2 Which ONE of the following statements about malignant melanoma in the UK is TRUE?
A It is increasing in incidence
B It is more common before puberty than after puberty
C It is more common in males than females
D Malignant melanomas are invariably pigmented
E The 2-year survival in metastatic melanoma is over 50%

13.3 In which ONE of the following skin disorders would the presence of pigmentation within a lesion suggest an alternative diagnosis to the diagnoses suggested below?
A Benign melanocytic naevus
B Malignant melanoma
C Guttate psoriasis
D Dermatofibroma
E Basal cell carcinoma

13.4 A 25-year-old woman with eczema has been using topical corticosteroid therapy on a daily basis for 6 months prior to presentation. Which ONE of the following findings suggests an alternative explanation to that of an adverse drug effect resulting from corticosteroid therapy?
A Dermal atrophy most marked in the face and body folds
B Striae, particularly in the body folds
C Suppression of the hypothalamo–pituitary–adrenal axis
D Decreased hair growth
E Spread of skin infection

13.5 A 35-year-old laboratory technician presents with an intensely itchy, papulosquamous rash affecting the hands and upper limbs. The social and occupational history has identified a number of potential sensitizing agents in the development of his contact eczema. Which ONE of the following factors can be discounted as a likely sensitizing factor?
A Aluminium measuring rule
B Sticking plasters
C Lanolin ointment
D Rubber shoes
E Epoxy resin glue

13.6 In evaluating a widespread scaly rash of sudden onset, which ONE of the following statements is TRUE?
A A slowly-progressive course from late adolescence suggests atopic eczema
B Involvement of elbow and knee flexure surfaces suggests psoriasis
C Onset in the scalp suggests pityriasis rosea
D Absence of itch suggests pityriasis versicolor
E Absence of itch suggests lichen planus

13.7 Which ONE of the statements about skin disorders is TRUE?
A Pemphigus vulgaris is more likely to develop in patients with pernicious anaemia
B Crohn's disease may present with dermatitis herpetiformis
C Lichen planus typically produces a periumbilical rash
D Pemphigus vulgaris is characterized by an intraepidermal blistering eruption
E Bullous pemphigoid is likely to respond to a gluten-free diet

13.8 A 34-year-old garage mechanic presents with an acneiform rash over the face and thorax. The previous history includes manic depression and asthma. Which ONE of the following factors can be discounted as a likely contributory agent in the evolution of his skin eruption?
A Exposure to chlorinated hydrocarbons
B Corticosteroid therapy
C Androgenic steroid therapy
D Lithium carbonate therapy
E Amoxicillin therapy

13.9 In a patient who has observed an increasing tendency to develop a deep suntan on minimal exposure to the sun, which ONE of the following factors can be discounted as a likely cause of the hyperpigmentation?
A Amiodarone therapy
B Chlorpromazine therapy
C Phenytoin therapy
D Mepacrine therapy
E Haemochromatosis

13.10 Which ONE of the following findings suggests an alternative diagnosis to lichen planus?
A   Involvement of the skin, nails, hair and mucous membranes
B   Dense subepidermal lymphocytic infiltration on histology
C   Itchy, purplish, polygonal, shiny skin papules
D   Hyperpigmentation at sites of previous lesions
E   Complete resolution following topical steroid therapy

13.11 Which ONE of the following suggests an alternative diagnosis to erythema multiforme?
A   Target-like skin lesions of the hands and feet
B   Skin eruption lasting 1–2 weeks
C   Absence of vesiculation or blistering
D   Involvement of the eyes, genitalia and mouth
E   Association with underlying systemic malignancy

13.12 Which ONE of the following features is MOST consistent with the diagnosis of erythema nodosum?
A   The presence of non-tender nodules over the shins
B   Lesions which disappear after 7–10 days
C   The presence of fever, malaise and polyarthralgia
D   The development of oral and genital mucosal ulceration
E   A tendency to affect the elderly more than younger subjects

13.13 Which ONE of the following features is MOST consistent with a diagnosis of seborrhoeic keratosis?
A   Appearance before the age of 30 years
B   Discrete irregular lesions in light-exposed skin areas
C   Yellow-brown, pedunculated lesions on the trunk or face
D   Lesions developing at the site of previous skin trauma
E   Eventual transition to squamous cell carcinoma

13.14 Which ONE of the following statements about systemic disorders affecting the nails is TRUE?
A   Koilonychia suggests the presence of molybdenum deficiency
B   Onycholysis is typically associated with iron deficiency
C   Leuconychia is associated with reversal of the plasma albumin/globulin ratio
D   Splinter haemorrhages invariably indicate the presence of infective endocarditis
E   Beau's lines appear synchronously on both the finger-and toenails

13.15 A 19-year-old woman presents with a rash limited to the scalp. In which ONE of the following disorders is scalp involvement typical of the condition?
A   Systemic lupus erythematosus
B   Scabies
C   Tylosis
D   Psoriasis
E   Erythrasma

13.16 Which ONE of the following features best characterizes severe exfoliative dermatitis?
A Absence of hypoalbuminaemia
B Presence of vesicles
C Atopic eczema is a predisposing condition
D Systemic corticosteroid therapy is contraindicated
E Absence of a past history of psoriasis

13.17 Which ONE of the following skin disorders is MOST likely to be associated with an underlying visceral malignancy?
A Erythema multiforme
B Pityriasis versicolor
C Dermatographia
D Acanthosis nigricans
E Guttate psoriasis

13.18 Which ONE of the following statements about dermatitis herpetiformis is TRUE?
A Uninvolved skin exhibits IgA deposits at the dermo-epidermal junction
B There is 90% chance of spontaneous remission
C Dapsone treatment typically causes a megaloblastic anaemia
D The mucous membranes are characteristically spared
E Partial or total villous atrophy occurs in 10–20% of patients

13.19 In which ONE of the following disorders would the development of blistering skin lesions suggest an alternative diagnosis?
A Psoriasis
B Acute intermittent porphyria
C Allergic contact dermatitis
D Rosacea
E Pityriasis versicolor

13.20 In which ONE of the following disorders would the development of cutaneous ulceration suggest an alternative diagnosis?
A Polyarteritis nodosa
B Dermatitis artefacta
C Rheumatoid arthritis
D Sickle-cell anaemia
E Lupus pernio

ANSWERS

13.1   A   ✔   Asymmetry
        B   ✘   Border
        C   ✘   Colour
        D   ✘   Diameter
        E   ✘   Elevation (viz. the ABCDE rule)

13.2   A   ✔   Doubled in the past 10 years
        B   ✘   Rare before puberty
        C   ✘   Female to male ratio is 2:1
        D   ✘   Truly amelanotic lesions are rare
        E   ✘   <10% survive in stage III

13.3   A   ✘
        B   ✘   Important in the differential diagnosis
        C   ✔
        D   ✘   Typically on the extremities of young adults
        E   ✘   Usually facial in site

13.4   A   ✘   There may also be purpura
        B   ✘   The skin is thin and fragile
        C   ✘   Systemic absorption can occur
        D   ✔   Hirsutism may rarely occur
        E   ✘   Local and systemic immune function may be compromised

13.5   A   ✔   Nickel is the metal most likely to cause a problem
        B   ✘   Colophony in sticking plaster
        C   ✘   Due to wool alcohols
        D   ✘   Or rubber clothing
        E   ✘   And other resins

13.6   A   ✘   Often starts in the first 2 years of life
        B   ✘   Involvement of extensor surfaces suggests psoriasis
        C   ✘   Suggests psoriasis
        D   ✔   In contrast to eczema
        E   ✘   Intensely itchy

13.7   A   ✘
        B   ✘   Coeliac disease
        C   ✘   Lichen planus typically affects the volar aspect of the wrists
        D   ✔
        E   ✘   Dermatitis herpetiformis

13.8   A   ✘   Ducts may be obstructed
        B   ✘   Lesions elsewhere suggest an alternative diagnosis
        C   ✘   And oestrogenic therapy; antibiotics can be helpful
        D   ✘   Largely hormonally mediated
        E   ✔   Typically produces a maculopapulous erythematous rash

13.9   A   ✗   Slate grey in exposed areas
      B   ✗
      C   ✔
      D   ✗   Yellow pigmentation
      E   ✗   Due to melanin deposition

13.10   A   ✗   But the nails are usually normal
      B   ✗   With hyperkeratosis and basal cell degeneration
      C   ✗   Perhaps with Wickham's striae
      D   ✗   Post-inflammatory pigmentation is common
      E   ✔   But topical steroids may aid symptoms

13.11   A   ✗   'Bull's eye' lesions
      B   ✗   The eruption rapidly resolves
      C   ✔   Classical features of the condition
      D   ✗   May be severe systemic upset
      E   ✗   Radiotherapy may precipitate such lesions

13.12   A   ✗   Lesions are painful
      B   ✗   Resolve over several weeks leaving bruises
      C   ✔   Mild systemic upset is typical
      D   ✗   Suggests an alternative diagnosis
      E   ✗   More common in younger individuals

13.13   A   ✗   Tend to occur in later life
      B   ✗   Light exposure is not a factor
      C   ✔   Pedunculated or sessile
      D   ✗   Köbner phenomenon is typically seen in psoriasis
      E   ✗   Not pre-malignant

13.14   A   ✗   A feature of iron deficiency
      B   ✗   Psoriasis, also nail pitting and subungual hyperkeratosis
      C   ✔   Seen in advanced liver disease and nephrotic syndrome
      D   ✗   May be associated with trauma
      E   ✗   Greater speed of growth in the fingernails than the toenails

13.15   A   ✗   Discoid lupus erythematosus causes scarring alopecia
      B   ✗   Finger webs, wrists and genitalia. Scalp and face spared
      C   ✗   Confined to palms and soles
      D   ✔   Causes adherent scaling
      E   ✗   *Corynebacterium minutissimum* infection affects toes, axillae and groins

13.16   A   ✗   Serum albumin falls due to skin loss and reduced protein synthesis
      B   ✗   Usually absent; redness, itch, oedema, scaling and heat predominate
      C   ✔
      D   ✗   May be life-saving
      E   ✗   Previous psoriasis is an aetiological factor

13.17 A ✗ Infection, drugs, collagen, vascular diseases are the causes
       B ✗ Commensal yeast infection
       C ✗ Usually associated with urticaria
       D ✔ Gastric adenocarcinoma or lymphoma especially
       E ✗ Exacerbations may be associated with alcohol abuse

13.18 A ✔ Usually IgA predominates
       B ✗ Chronic disorder
       C ✗ Causes haemolytic anaemia
       D ✗ Typically involved
       E ✗ Occurs in 80–90%

13.19 A ✗ Papulo-squamous eruption
       B ✗ Unlike porphyria cutanea tarda which often affects exposed areas of skin
       C ✔ Healing to leave scars
       D ✗
       E ✗

13.20 A ✗ Due to cutaneous vasculitis
       B ✗ Self-inflicted skin lesion with irregular, bizarre configurations
       C ✗ Especially Felty's syndrome
       D ✗ Usually on lower limbs
       E ✔ Dusky infiltrated plaques on nose and fingers in sarcoidosis

14

Ophthalmology

14.1 In an 81-year-old man who presents with a painless and
progressive loss of vision bilaterally, which ONE of the following
disorders is the MOST likely diagnosis?
A Central retinal artery occlusion
B Retinitis pigmentosa
C Senile macular degeneration
D Cranial arteritis
E Retinoblastoma

14.2 An 18-year-old woman returning from travelling through Central
America presents with unilateral, painless orbital oedema
without visual loss or diplopia. Which ONE of the following
disorders is the MOST likely diagnosis?
A Third cranial nerve palsy
B Cavernous sinus thrombosis
C *Trypanosoma cruzi* infection
D Hypoparathyroidism
E Hereditary angio-oedema

14.3 A 60-year-old man presents with visual loss and is suspected of
having chronic simple (open-angle) glaucoma. On examination,
which ONE of the following features is MOST likely to be
present?
A A painful red eye
B Papilloedema
C Diminished peripheral vision
D Absence of cupping of optic disc
E An asymmetrical quadrantanopia

14.4 Following a febrile illness, a 22-year-old woman in the second
trimester of pregnancy presents with blurred vision. On
ophthalmoscopy, there is evidence of choroiditis. Which ONE of
the following infectious diseases is LEAST likely to be
responsible?
A Gonorrhoea
B Histoplasmosis
C Toxoplasmosis
D Cytomegalovirus infection
E Tuberculosis

14.5 Which ONE of the following disorders typically causes an acute anterior uveitis?
A Systemic lupus erythematosus
B Sarcoidosis
C Herpes simplex infection
D Whipple's disease
E Toxocariasis

14.6 Which ONE of the following disorders is typically associated with soft retinal exudates?
A HIV infection
B Central retinal vein thrombosis
C Early diabetic retinopathy
D Marfan's syndrome
E Vitamin A deficiency

14.7 In which ONE of the following lesions would a right homonymous hemianopia be MOST likely to occur?
A The left optic tract
B The temporal division of the left optic radiation
C The optic chiasma
D The right lateral geniculate body
E The left optic nerve

14.8 Which ONE of the following features would be an EXPECTED finding following infarction of the third cranial nerve in a patient with cavernous sinus thrombosis?
A Paralysis of abduction of the eye
B Absence of facial sweating
C Partial ptosis of the eye
D Pupillary constriction
E Absence of the accommodation reflex

14.9 Which ONE of the following features would be an EXPECTED finding associated with paralysis of the fourth cranial nerve?
A Weakness of the inferior oblique muscle
B Pupillary dilatation
C Impaired downward gaze in abduction
D Elevation and abduction of the eye
E Nystagmus more marked in the abducted eye

14.10 Which ONE of the following disorders would BEST explain the absence of pupillary constriction in either eye on shining a light into the right pupil?
A Bilateral Argyll Robertson pupils
B Unilateral right-sided, Holmes–Adie pupil
C Left optic nerve lesion
D Right oculomotor nerve lesion
E Bilateral Horner's syndrome

ANSWERS

14.1 A ✗ Sudden loss of vision
      B ✗ Onset under the age of 20 years
      C ✔
      D ✗ Sudden irreversible blindness
      E ✗ 90% present under the age of 3 years

14.2 A ✗ Ptosis but not oedema
      B ✗ No evidence of 3,4,5 cranial nerve involvement
      C ✔ Romana's sign in S. American trypanosomiasis transmitted by the reduviid bug
      D ✗ Although cataracts occur in this condition
      E ✗ Previous episodes and typically bilateral

14.3 A ✗ Suggests acute, closed-angle glaucoma
      B ✗ Often optic atrophy
      C ✔ Characteristic
      D ✗ Often present
      E ✗ This would suggest a lesion of the optic tract

14.4 A ✔ Usually associated with an anterior uveitis
      B ✗ More likely to cause a posterior rather than anterior uveitis
      C ✗
      D ✗ Also other infections including syphilis
      E ✗ Choroidal tubercles heal producing choroiditis

14.5 A ✗ Scleritis and episcleritis
      B ✔
      C ✗ Herpes zoster infection
      D ✗ Papillitis or choroiditis
      E ✗ Low-grade posterior uveitis

14.6 A ✔ Cotton wool spots occur in many stages of HIV disease
      B ✗ Causes retinal haemorrhages
      C ✗ Indicates advanced retinal ischaemia
      D ✗ Dislocated lens is usual eye feature
      E ✗ Keratomalacia

14.7 A ✔ The optic tract runs between optic chiasma and lateral geniculate body
      B ✗ Produces an upper quadrantanopic field defect
      C ✗ Midline lesions cause bitemporal hemianopia
      D ✗ Left lateral geniculate body
      E ✗ Left monocular visual loss

14.8 A ✗ Suggests sixth cranial nerve palsy
      B ✗ Occurs in Horner's syndrome
      C ✗ Complete paralysis of levator palpebrae superioris
      D ✗ Pupillary dilatation due to impaired parasympathetic tone
      E ✔ And absence of the direct light response

14.9   A ✗ Superior oblique
        B ✗ No pupillary change
        C ✗ Impaired downward gaze in adduction
        D ✔ Head may tilt towards normal side
        E ✗ Suggests an internuclear ophthalmoplegia

14.10   A ✔ Accommodation preserved
        B ✗ Consensual response would be present; the defect is in
               the ciliary ganglia
        C ✗ An afferent defect in the right eye
        D ✗ Only the reaction in right eye would be impaired
        E ✗ Both pupils may be small but responsive

Index